100 Questions & Answers About Pancreatic Cancer

Eileen O'Reilly, MD
Joanne Frankel Kelvin, RN, MSN

JONES AND BARTLETT PUBLISHERS

Sudbury, Massachusetts

BOSTON   TORONTO   LONDON   SINGAPORE

World Headquarters
Jones and Bartlett
Publishers
40 Tall Pine Drive
Sudbury, MA 01776
info@jbpub.com
www.jbpub.com

Jones and Bartlett
Publishers Canada
2406 Nikanna Road
Mississauga, ON L5C
2W6
CANADA

Jones and Bartlett
Publishers International
Barb House, Barb Mews
London W6 7PA
UK

Library of Congress Cataloging-in-Publication Data

O'Reilly, Eileen.
    100 questions & answers about pancreatic cancer / Eileen O'Reilly,
Joanne Frankel Kelvin.
        p. cm.
Includes index.
    ISBN 0-7637-2057-7
    1. Pancreas--Cancer--Popular works.   I. Title: One hundred questions
and answers about pancreatic cancer.   II. Kelvin, Joanne Frankel.   III.
Title.
    RC280.P25 O745 2003
    616.99'437--dc21

                                                        2002152131

The authors, editor, and publisher have made every effort to provide accurate information. However, they are not responsible for errors, omissions, or for any outcomes related to the use of the contents of this book and take no responsibility for the use of the products described. Treatments and side effects described in this book may not be applicable to all patients; likewise, some patients may require a dose or experience a side effect that is not described herein. The reader should confer with his or her own physician regarding specific treatments and side effects. Drugs and medical devices are discussed that may have limited availability or be controlled by the Food and Drug Administration (FDA) for use only in a research study or clinical trial. The drug information presented has been derived from reference sources, recently published data, and pharmaceutical research data. Research, clinical practice, and government regulations often change the accepted standard in this field. When consideration is being given to use of any drug in the clinical setting, the health care provider or reader is responsible for determining FDA status of the drug, reading the package insert, reviewing prescribing information for the most up-to-date recommendations on dose, precautions, and contraindications, and determining the appropriate usage for the product. This is especially important in the case of drugs that are new or seldom used. The statements of patients quoted in this book represent their own opinions and do not necessarily reflect the views of the authors or the publisher.

Acquisitions Editor: Christopher Davis
Production Editor: Elizabeth Platt
Cover Design: Philip Regan
Manufacturing Buyer: Therese Bräuer
Composition: Northeast Compositors
Printing and Binding: Malloy Lithographing
Cover Printer: Malloy Lithographing

Printed in the United States of America
07 06 05 04 03   10 9 8 7 6 5 4 3 2 1

Contents

- What can I do to prevent or relieve nausea and vomiting related to my chemotherapy or radiation therapy?
- I was told that chemotherapy may cause a drop in my blood counts. What does this mean?
- I have difficulty sleeping at night. What can I do to sleep better and feel more rested?
- Will I have pain? What options are available for treating my pain?
- I never feel hungry and am concerned about losing weight. What can I do to increase my appetite and maintain my weight?

Howard Simon, Pancreatic Cancer Patient
July 2002

January 11, 2001, was my 54th birthday—and the day exploratory surgery confirmed the preliminary diagnosis that I had received ten days earlier. I had pancreatic cancer that had metastasized to my liver. What do I do? Where do I go from here? How long do I have to live? What treatments are available to me? My wife ... my children ... I needed information; I wanted answers!

I first entered my local hospital on New Year's Day, jaundiced and in pain. The doctors suspected gall bladder disease or hepatitis, but a computed tomography scan showed otherwise. My wife and I spent the next ten days crying and in shock, waiting to go into Memorial Sloan-Kettering for a second opinion. After confirming the diagnosis of metastatic pancreatic cancer, the surgeon strongly recommended that we speak with Dr. Eileen O'Reilly, an oncologist who was conducting a clinical trial pairing gemcitibine, the standard drug used to treat pancreatic cancer, with DX8951f, an experimental drug.

Dr. O'Reilly was forthright in our first meeting, telling me about my treatment options. How were my wife and I supposed to make such a life and death decision? We certainly didn't feel knowledgeable enough! We only knew that we were determined to fight this disease as aggressively as we could, and we therefore opted to participate in Dr. O'Reilly's clinical trial. I began treatment on February 14th, 2001, and during the past 17 months, my condition has remained amazingly stable.

Educating myself about this disease has not been an easy process. Immediately after diagnosis I realized that little information was available to patients, not only about the disease itself but also about treatment options (clinical trials) and their side effects and about ways of addressing the psychological and emotional turmoil one finds oneself in. In addition, in order for me to feel peace of mind with regard to the future of my family, I needed guidance in putting my affairs in order.

In the many months that I have been undergoing chemotherapy, I have talked with so many patients who, like myself, lack critical information about pancreatic cancer. Not having adequate information limits our ability to formulate the right questions to pose to our doctors.

Dr. Eileen O'Reilly and Registered Nurse Joanne Frankel Kelvin have done a magnificent job of formulating and then responding to many of the questions that a pancreatic cancer patient could have. This book provides patients and their families with the much needed information and direction that are so vital to their understanding of and ability to cope with this horrific disease. This book should be required reading for all pancreatic cancer patients and their families.

Mr. Howard Simon is 55 years old and has metastatic pancreatic cancer involving the liver. He was originally diagnosed in December 2000. He is receiving chemotherapy as part of a clinical trial, which he joined in February 2001. He has had excellent control of his cancer while on this chemotherapy regimen, and he currently continues this same treatment—now approaching the 18-month mark. In addition, he continues to enjoy a very productive professional and personal life despite his diagnosis and treatment.

From the moment that a person receives a diagnosis of cancer, he or she embarks on a journey filled with confusing road signs, unexpected detours, and an uncertain destination. For patients with pancreatic cancer, this journey is particularly challenging because the prognosis is poor. About 30,000 people in the United States and 175,000 worldwide are diagnosed each year with pancreatic cancer. Unfortunately, most people have advanced disease and are at a point at which the cancer is inoperable; however, it is important to recognize that most people diagnosed with this disease can be helped in both quality and length of life.

Until recently, pancreatic cancer received little public, medical, or federal attention. That is now changing, and with the efforts of patient support and research organizations (such as PanCan and the Lustgarten Foundation), the profile of pancreatic cancer is being elevated, and there is recognition that major innovations are urgently needed to have a meaningful impact on the outcome of this disease. In 2002, there was a large increase in federal research funding for pancreatic cancer; however, this still falls significantly behind that provided for other major cancers. We are grateful to Jones and Bartlett for recognizing the need to offer a source of information and support for patients with this disease.

We hope that this book will serve as a roadmap and guide to accompany you on the journey ahead. Specifically, we hope to provide you with information about the disease and its treatment, clarify issues as you make decisions about your care, help you manage the symptoms of the disease and side effects of treatment, and improve your ability to cope with the emotional and practical concerns that will come up for you and your family.

Eileen O'Reilly is a medical oncologist at Memorial Sloan-Kettering Cancer Center and has a major clinical and research interest in pancreatic cancer. Her work has focused on developing new therapies for this disease, including chemotherapeutic agents, vaccine strategies, and combinations of radiation therapy and cytostatic or targeted therapy drugs. She currently is helping to coordinate a large international clinical trial for advanced pancreatic cancer. Her other areas of interest are the genetics of pancreatic cancer, the associations of pancreatic cancer with other malignancies, and issues related to screening and early detection. She is indebted to Mr. Howard Simon, a gentleman with metastatic pancreatic cancer who is currently receiving chemotherapy. His insight, intelligence, and personal experience have greatly added to the depth and breadth of this book.

Joanne Frankel Kelvin is an oncology nurse at Memorial Sloan-Kettering Cancer Center, recently collaborating with Eileen O'Reilly in caring for patients with pancreatic cancer. She has been a nurse for over 25 years, specializing in oncology nursing for most of that time. The courage, strength, and love of her patients and their families have inspired her. She dedicates this book to them with gratitude for all that they have taught her over the years. In addition, she thanks Eileen O'Reilly for offering her the opportunity to coauthor this book and her husband for his constant support.

Eileen O'Reilly, MD
Joanne Frankel Kelvin, RN, MSN

Jones and Bartlett Publishers also thank the patient contributors, Joy McCully and John Harty, for the time they took to read and comment on this book. Their contributions are invaluable.

PART ONE

The Basics

What is cancer?

What is the pancreas gland, and where is it located?

What does my pancreas gland do?

More ...

1. What is cancer?

Cells

the smallest structural unit of a living organism

Cancer is the growth and division of **cells** in an unregulated fashion. Normally, orderly signals control cells and indicate when they should grow and divide. We call this natural turnover the "cell cycle." Normal cells are usually in a resting phase of the cell cycle—performing their usual functions. They grow and divide only when natural chemical "messengers" in the body tell them to do so, and they stop growing and die when internal regulatory mechanisms indicate. Cells become

Cancerous

malignant, capable of invading tissue and spreading to distant organs

cancerous when the regulatory mechanisms that control cell growth don't work, such as when the normal control points in the cell cycle are turned off or restrained. They continue to grow uncontrollably, eventually forming a malignant **tumor** or mass of can-

Tumor

abnormal growth, can be cancerous (malignant) or noncancerous (benign)

cerous cells within an organ. These cells can interrupt the normal function of the organ or system in which they form by crowding out normal cells or blocking passageways from one organ to another (e.g., when a tumor of the digestive tract blocks food from passing through the intestine). Unlike normal cells, cancer cells also have the ability to invade other organs directly or to spread via the blood stream and **lym-**

Lymphatic channels

vessels throughout the body that conduct lymph fluid

phatic channels to other areas of the body, a process called **metastasis** (see Question 15).

Metastasis

spread of a malignant tumor to a distant organ

The origin of the cancer is the primary site (thus, "pancreatic cancer" starts off in the pancreas). Secondary sites, or metastases, are the places to where the cancer has spread. Regardless of the site of spread, a cancer is always referred to by the primary site of origin (e.g., pancreas cancer spread to the lung is called metastatic pancreatic cancer and not lung cancer). Knowing the original location of the cancer is important because different cancers respond to different treatments; for example, a drug that works well on lung cancer may not work at all on a pancreatic cancer that has moved to the lung.

2. What is the pancreas gland, and where is it located?

Your pancreas gland is an organ that is located in the back of the upper abdomen near the backbone (Figure 1). It is tucked in between your small bowel (duodenum) and stomach, which sits in front of the gland. It consists of a head, body, and tail (Figure 2). The major portion of the pancreas (head) is situated in the center of the abdomen, with the body and tail extending over to the left side of the abdomen at the back. The gland measures approximately 6 to 8 inches. The pancreatic duct, a major drainage channel for pancreatic secretions, runs through the length of the gland and empties pancreatic secretions into the small bowel. The common bile duct, the drainage channel from the gallbladder, runs through the head of the pancreas and joins the pancreatic duct to form the ampulla of Vater before it empties into the small bowel. Pancreatic cancers that arise in the head of the pancreas commonly cause **jaundice** (yellowing of the skin and eyes) because growth of the cancer blocks the bile duct. Your pancreatic gland is essential to life and has several important functions that are detailed in the next question.

3. What does my pancreas gland do?

Your pancreas gland has several major roles that are divided into **endocrine** and **exocrine** functions. The major endocrine role is the control of blood sugar, and the major exocrine function is to make digestive enzymes. The Islet cells, which are in the tail of the

Jaundice

yellowing of the skin or eyes from a build up of bilirubin in the blood stream

Endocrine

gland that secretes substances directly into the blood stream

Exocrine

gland that secretes substances through a duct

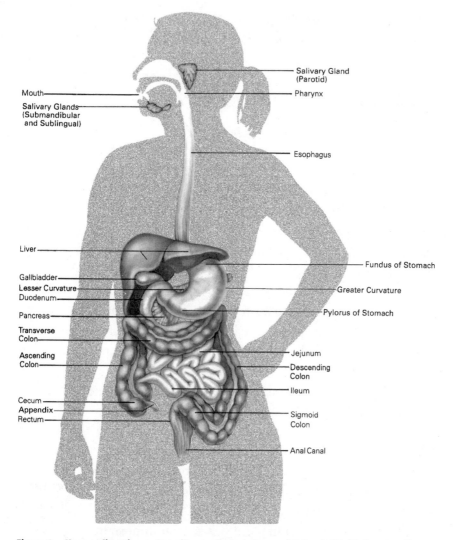

Mouth

Salivary Glands
(Submandibular
and Sublingual)

Salivary Gland
(Parotid)

Pharynx

Esophagus

Liver

Gallbladder
Lesser Curvature
Duodenum

Pancreas

Transverse
Colon

Ascending
Colon

Cecum
Appendix
Rectum

Fundus of Stomach

Greater Curvature

Pylorus of Stomach

Jejunum

Descending
Colon

Ileum

Sigmoid
Colon

Anal Canal

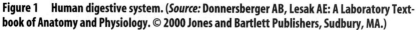

Figure 1   Human digestive system. (*Source:* Donnersberger AB, Lesak AE: A Laboratory Textbook of Anatomy and Physiology. © 2000 Jones and Bartlett Publishers, Sudbury, MA.)

pancreas, produce insulin, a hormone that controls the blood sugar level. Insulin production is often affected when pancreatic cancer is present, usually leading to higher blood sugar levels or frank diabetes. The reasons for high blood sugar levels in patients with pancreatic cancer are not entirely clear. It is thought that

The Basics

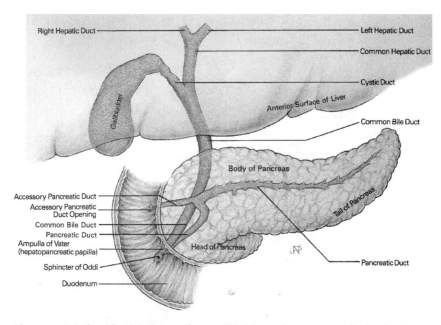

Right Hepatic Duct

Left Hepatic Duct

Common Hepatic Duct

Cystic Duct

Gallbladder

Anterior Surface of Liver

Common Bile Duct

Body of Pancreas

Tail of Pancreas

Accessory Pancreatic Duct

Accessory Pancreatic Duct Opening

Common Bile Duct

Pancreatic Duct

Ampulla of Vater (hepatopancreatic papilla)

Head of Pancreas

Pancreatic Duct

Sphincter of Oddi

Duodenum

Figure 2   Relationship of the human liver, gallbladder, and pancrease to the duodenum. (*Source:* Donnersberger AB, Lesak AE: A Laboratory Textbook of Anatomy and Physiology. © 2000 Jones and Bartlett Publishers, Sudbury, MA. Drawing by P.J. Nicholls.)

certain substances that make insulin less effective are circulating in the blood stream at higher levels in pancreatic cancer patients compared with people who do not have pancreatic cancer.

The second major function of the pancreas gland is production and secretion of digestive enzymes into the duodenum (small bowel). Food breakdown and absorption are often disturbed when you have pancreatic cancer, partly because the main pancreatic duct or drainage channel is blocked and also because of inadequate production and secretion of pancreatic enzymes. With pancreatic cancer, you may have symptoms such as gas, bloating, oily fatty bowel movements, and weight loss, which you can correct by taking supplemental pancreatic enzymes (see Question 61).

4. Are there different types of pancreatic cancer?

Yes. Pancreatic cancer can be broken down into exocrine and endocrine types. Pancreatic cancer typically refers to pancreatic adenocarcinoma (also known as ductal adenocarcinoma), which involves the exocrine portion of the pancreas. Ductal adenocarcinomas arise mostly in the head of the gland (70%), but they also appear in the body (20%) and tail (10%). In this book, we primarily refer to adenocarcinomas of the pancreas, which account for more than 90% of all types of pancreatic cancers. Another type of pancreatic cancer is endocrine pancreatic cancer, also known as neuroendocrine cancer. These cancers usually arise in the body and tail of the pancreas and generally grow slowly, consequently having a better **prognosis**. Lymphomas and sarcomas also rarely occur in the pancreas. Lymphomas and sarcomas of the pancreas are treated the same as if they were located elsewhere in the body.

Prognosis
the most likely outcome of a disease

5. Who gets pancreatic cancer, and how many people are diagnosed each year?

If you are male, African American, more than 60 years old, or a heavy smoker, you are at a higher risk for developing pancreatic cancer. The biggest single changeable risk factor for developing pancreatic cancer is smoking, which increases your risk of developing pancreatic cancer approximately twofold and probably accounts for approximately 40% of all pancreatic cancers. Other risk factors for developing pancreatic cancer include a high-

The biggest single changeable risk factor for developing pancreatic cancer is smoking.

The Basics

fat, low-fiber diet, heavy alcohol use, and jobs that involve regular contact with chemicals, toxic metals, or gas. In total, these latter risk factors contribute a relatively small proportion of the risk. A personal or family history of pancreatic cancer is one of your most important and unalterable risk factors for developing pancreatic cancer. Approximately 10% of all pancreatic cancers have a **hereditary** or **genetic** component. We increasingly recognize that certain genetic **mutations** predispose to the development of pancreatic cancer and associate pancreatic cancer with other cancers. For example, pancreatic cancer may be associated with malignant melanoma; breast, prostate, and colon cancer; and certain types of leukemia and brain cancers. The association of diabetes mellitus (Type II) with pancreatic cancer is controversial. There are multiple studies assessing the exact relationship between the two. The current thinking is that diabetes and chronic pancreatitis (a long-standing inflammatory condition of the pancreas, often attributed to alcohol) are associated but do not have a cause and effect relationship. Other traditionally quoted risk factors (e.g., coffee use) have been discounted in recent times.

In the United States, the incidence of pancreatic cancer has slowly been increasing over the last several decades. We anticipate that approximately 30,000 people will be diagnosed this year in the United States, and approximately 175,000 cases will be diagnosed worldwide. Many people believe that the latter figure is a significant underestimate of the total burden of disease, as pancreatic cancer can be difficult to diagnose—and in many developing countries, it may never be diagnosed. When you look at the rate of pancreatic cancer in another way, approximately 8 to 12 per

Hereditary
passed on through the genes from one generation to the next

Genetic
affected by genes, parts of chromosomes which influence the structure or function of the body

Mutations
abnormal alteration in the structure of the DNA molecule (gene)

The incidence of pancreatic cancer has slowly been increasing over the last several decades.

100,000 of the population develop this disease, and worldwide it is the 13th most common cancer in terms of frequency and the 9th leading cause of cancer-related deaths. Overall, pancreatic cancer accounts for approximately 2% of all cancer diagnoses.

6. Does pancreatic cancer run in families?

Yes. Pancreatic cancer is increasingly recognized as having a significant familial component—that is, heredity contributes to its development. This is the case for approximately 10% to 15% of patients with pancreatic cancer. Several genes have been identified that contribute to the risk of developing pancreatic cancer; however, for most of the familial risk, the offending gene(s) has not yet been identified.

Heredity contributes to its development.

Five or six well-recognized genetic syndromes are associated with pancreatic cancer. A rare but important one is hereditary pancreatitis, which results from a single gene abnormality that causes destruction of the pancreatic gland by unchecked activity of digestive enzymes. Family members who carry this genetic mutation have a 40% to 70% lifetime chance of developing pancreatic cancer and often do so by their 40s. A more common genetic syndrome that is associated with pancreatic cancer is hereditary nonpolyposis coli. In certain families that have a mutation in the *p16* gene, pancreatic cancer may occur in association with malignant melanoma. The major implication of these genetic syndromes is not that screening for pancreatic cancer is possible (at this time it is not) but that screening may be appropriate for the associated cancers.

The National Familial Pancreatic Tumor Registry (*www.pathology.jhu.edu/pancreas*) was set up in 1994 to better estimate the risk of familial pancreatic cancer. You, your family members, and your physician are allowed to register as part of this database. More than 700–800 families have been enrolled. An early assessment of this database indicates that for healthy family members with two or more first-degree relatives (sibling, parent, child) with pancreatic cancer, the personal risk of developing the disease is 18-fold higher than in the general population. For healthy individuals with three or more first-degree relatives with the disease, the personal risk is an amazing 57-fold higher than the general population.

7. Are other cancers associated with pancreatic cancer?

Yes. Pancreatic cancer is associated with several different malignancies. As noted in the previous question, this disease may be associated with malignant melanoma via the *p21* gene. In families with hereditary nonpolyposis coli, pancreatic cancer may occur in association with colorectal, breast, prostate, stomach, and endometrial cancers.

8. Are there any ways of preventing pancreatic cancer?

Possibly. Some of the lifestyle behaviors that you can change to decrease your risk for developing pancreatic cancer are stopping smoking, eating a low-fat, high-fiber diet, and minimizing alcohol consumption. These may be particularly important if your family has a hereditary tendency for pancreatic cancer. It is important to recognize that for most people who develop this disease, no way of preventing the disease is currently known. Again, quitting smoking is a key public health measure that may influence the overall frequency of this cancer and may possibly also decrease the personal risk of developing this disease.

9. How long do people live after they have been diagnosed with pancreatic cancer?

The life expectancy of a person diagnosed with pancreatic cancer is directly related to the stage at diagnosis. For example, people who have operable pancreatic cancer do significantly better than patients with bulky metastatic disease (disease that has spread to other organs). On average, the estimated survival for an individual who has had a potentially curative operation for pancreatic cancer (e.g., **Whipple surgery**) is approximately 13 to 20 months. For individuals with metastatic disease, the average survival is 3 to 9 months, and for individuals with inoperable but localized pancreatic cancer, the estimated survival is approximately 6 to 12 months. These figures refer to populations of people and not to individuals. Therefore, the actual life expectancy for a given person can be significantly greater or less than the average.

Whipple surgery

surgical removal of the head of the pancreas, the upper end of the duodenum, and the lower end of the bile duct; also involves reconnecting the stomach, the bile duct, and the pancreatic duct to the small intestine.

10. What are some of the misconceptions about pancreatic cancer?

Pancreatic cancer is often thought to be an untreatable and rapidly fatal disease. Although this may be true for some patients, it is important to recognize that most people diagnosed with this disease can be helped, sometimes significantly, in both quality and length of life. Traditionally and all too typically, there has been

Most people diagnosed with this disease can be helped in both quality and length of life.

an approach to treating this disease in which doctors and patients alike shrug their shoulders and accept the idea that the patient is doomed. Thankfully, with education, distribution of information, and the introduction of new drugs for advanced disease, pancreatic cancer is increasingly being recognized as a treatable disease. One of the most important recent developments has been the licensure of gemcitabine (Gemzar) for patients with inoperable pancreatic cancer. This has set off much worldwide interest in looking at this disease from a basic science viewpoint through to clinical therapeutics. Thankfully now too, increasing amounts of federal, charitable, and industry money are being directed toward pancreatic research.

Pancreatic cancer is increasingly being recognized as a treatable disease.

The Basics

PART TWO

Diagnosis and Staging

What are the symptoms of pancreatic cancer?

How is pancreatic cancer diagnosed, and what tests are used in confirming the diagnosis?

What is a pathology report, and what can I learn from it?

More ...

11. What are the symptoms of pancreatic cancer?

Joy's Comment:

I had upper abdominal pain for about 4 months before it was diagnosed as pancreatic cancer. I lost weight because I noticed a correlation between eating and the onset of pain. The doctors thought it was reflux and did an upper gastrointestinal exam and colonoscopy before finally doing a computed tomography (CT) scan, which found the tumor. I had no particular increase in fatigue and no other symptoms. I had a 3-cm tumor at the head of the pancreas with no spread to any lymph nodes or organs.

The symptoms of pancreatic cancer may be variable and are often nonspecific, thus representing a variety of possibilities besides pancreatic cancer. Typically, dark urine, pale bowel movements, itching, and jaundice may show the development of pancreatic cancer. These latter symptoms usually come from a tumor arising in the head of the pancreas, causing blockage of the common bile duct (the drainage entrance from the liver to the small bowel, which passes through the head of the pancreas gland). Sometimes patients develop a loss of appetite, weight loss, tiredness, and decreased energy. If the tumor is advanced at the time of diagnosis, pain may be present. Pain may be located in the upper abdominal area or mid back or may sometimes be more spread out. Blood clots (**venous thromboses**) are strongly associated with pancreatic cancer, and may be the first symptom of the disease. **Migratory thrombophlebitis**, or transient superficial blood

Venous thrombosis
presence of a blood clot in a vein.

Migratory thrombophlebitis
formation of blood clots in the superficial veins of the arms or legs.

clots in the surface veins of the arms or legs, may also be associated with pancreatic cancer. As previously discussed, diabetes (Type II) has been associated with but does not appear to cause pancreatic cancer. If you develop diabetes at an older age and do not have a background of diabetes in your family, you should be assessed for the presence of pancreatic cancer. Often diabetes can come before the development of cancer by 6 to 18 months or longer, and sometimes diabetes develops after the disease has been diagnosed. The exact reasons for the development of diabetes are uncertain. It is not just a displacement situation, since the majority of pancreatic cancers are in the head of the gland and the majority of insulin-producing or Islet cells are in the tail of the gland.

If you develop diabetes at an older age and do not have a background of diabetes in your family, you should be assessed for the presence of pancreatic cancer.

12. How is pancreatic cancer diagnosed, and what tests are used in confirming the diagnosis?

Pancreatic cancer is diagnosed with good clinical insight and a variety of tests. Weight loss, decreased appetite, jaundice, and new diabetes should prompt suspicion for this disease. A high-quality **computed tomography (CT) scan** is probably the most useful test. When performed with oral and intravenous **contrast media**, it can show small tumors of the pancreas and whether the cancer has spread, for example, to the liver or the inner lining of the abdominal cavity (peritoneum). An **ultrasound** or **magnetic resonance**

Computed tomography (CT) scan
a diagnostic test that uses x-rays and a computer system to create detailed images of structures inside the body.

Contrast media
a substance given by mouth or by injection into a vein to provide better visualization of a particular organ on an x-ray or CT scan.

Ultrasound
a diagnostic test that uses sound waves to create images of structures inside the body.

Magnetic resonance imaging (MRI)

a diagnostic test that uses a large magnet, radio waves, and a computer system to create detailed images of structures inside the body.

Endoscopic retrograde cholangiopancreatogram (ERCP)

procedure done to evaluate the liver, gallbladder, bile ducts, and pancreas.

Ascites

abnormal build up of fluid in the abdominal cavity.

imaging (MRI)/cholangiopancreatography may provide additional or matching information. If you develop jaundice, an **endoscopic retrograde cholangiopancreatogram** (ERCP) may allow us to see the pancreatic and bile ducts. In addition, the latter test can allow placement of a stent, a plastic or metal tube that forces the bile duct open and lessens jaundice.

No specific blood tests are used to identify or check for pancreatic cancer. However, Ca19–9, a substance found on the surface of and shed by adenocarcinoma cells, may be seen and measured in the bloodstream in the majority of patients with pancreatic cancer. Ca19–9 can serve as a tumor marker because to some extent, following Ca19–9 levels can track the course of the disease. However, the levels may vary for many reasons aside from the activity of the cancer.

Sampling tissue from the pancreas itself (via a CT-guided biopsy) or taking scrapings from the lining of the pancreatic duct using an ERCP is usually needed to make the actual diagnosis of pancreatic cancer. Occasionally, in patients with metastatic disease involving the liver or with **ascites** (fluid) in the abdominal cavity, taking a liver biopsy or sampling the ascites helps to make a diagnosis. Sometimes the diagnosis is strongly suspected before an operation but is not confirmed until surgery is performed.

13. What is a pathology report, and what can I learn from it?

The pathology report describes important features of the cancer—specifically, the type of cancer (e.g., adenocarcinoma or neuroendocrine cancer). It also describes the degree of **differentiation** (how like or unlike the cancer cells are to normal pancreatic tissue). This may influence the prognosis. For patients who have undergone surgical removal of the cancer (e.g., Whipple surgery), the pathology report also describes several other features of the cancer:

- The number of lymph nodes removed is listed as well as the number of lymph nodes with cancerous cells.
- The edges (**margins**) of the cancer are described, specifically whether there is normal tissue surrounding the cancer on all sides. If not, microscopic cancer cells may be left behind.
- The tumor size, larger or smaller than 2 cm, is also included.

All of this information is important in determining the prognosis.

14. What is cancer staging, and why is it important?

Staging refers to the extent of the cancer. Most cancers, including pancreatic cancer, are staged with the T, N, M (tumor, node, metastases) classification. T refers to the tumor size. In pancreatic adenocarcinoma, this is described as being bigger or smaller than 2 cm. N refers to whether lymph nodes are (N1) or are not (N0) involved. M refers to the presence (M1) or absence (M0) of metastases. Operable pancreatic cancers are staged as I or II. Localized but inoperable pancreatic adenocarcinomas are staged as III, and metastatic pancreatic cancer (e.g., liver involvement) is staged as IV.

Differentiation

specialization in appearance and function.

Margins

the edges of any tissue removed by surgery.

Diagnosis and Staging

The importance of staging relates to the outcome of the cancer. As with other cancers, the earlier the stage, the better the outcome. For example, in a small, less than 2 cm, adenocarcinoma of the pancreas with no lymph nodes involved and clear edges—that is, T1, N0, M0, stage I—the estimated 5-year survival is approximately 40%. In contrast, for metastatic pancreatic cancer, M1 or stage IV, the estimated survival is 3 to 6 months; however, every case is different, and new treatments are becoming available all of the time.

The earlier the stage, the better the outcome.

15. What does metastatic mean? What does locally advanced mean? Where does pancreatic cancer spread to?

Pancreatic cancer most commonly spreads to the lymph nodes, liver, and abdominal cavity (peritoneum), although it can also spread to the lungs and the bones. When the peritoneum is involved, tumor cells are released into ascites. Sampling the fluid, if no previous diagnosis has been made, can establish metastatic cancer. Often the ascites accumulates to a significant extent, resulting in abdominal swelling, bloating, and weight gain. For comfort, the ascites can be drained via a bedside procedure called a **paracentesis**. With metastases, the cancer is difficult to treat and is inoperable, and thus, treatment (**chemotherapy**) is **palliative** (symptom relieving).

Locally advanced pancreatic cancer is diagnosed when pancreatic cancer is closely wrapped around major blood vessels. When this occurs, the cancer is inoperable, as these major blood vessels are essential for life and cannot be removed. In locally advanced pancreatic cancer, there is no metastases or spread

Paracentesis

procedure to drain fluid that has built up in the abdominal cavity.

Chemotherapy

medication used to destroy cancer cells.

Palliative

to relieve symptoms.

Locally advanced pancreatic cancer

stage of pancreatic cancer in which the tumor has invaded local tissue or is closely wrapped around vital structures, such as major blood vessels; can not be surgically removed.

(e.g., to the liver or the peritoneum); it is often treated with a combination of chemotherapy and radiation or sometimes chemotherapy alone. Occasionally, following combined chemotherapy and radiation for locally advanced disease, the cancer may shrink enough to become operable (resectable).

John's Comment:

When I was initially diagnosed, I was considered to be "borderline resectable." Although there were no indications that my cancer had spread to other organs, the CT image suggested that the tumor had wrapped around a major artery. After radiotherapy (10 doses over a 2-week period) and chemotherapy (Gemzar, one per week for 7 weeks) and allowing an additional 6 weeks to obtain the full benefit of these treatments, a CT scan showed that the tumor had been shrunk by over 50% and was clear of the artery. Was that ever good news!

PART THREE

Treatment

What methods are used to treat pancreatic cancer?

What is the difference between curative and palliative treatment?

What is performance status, and how does that influence my treatment choice?

More . . .

16. What methods are used to treat pancreatic cancer?

For any cancer, no matter the origin, you have three major options for treatment: surgery, radiation, and chemotherapy. If the pancreatic cancer is limited to a small area and is operable, then surgery is usually your first step. If surgery is successful, then you can use **adjuvant therapy** or postoperative chemotherapy and radiation combined to decrease the chance that the cancer will return.

Radiation is combined with chemotherapy for locally advanced pancreatic cancer (localized, but inoperable disease). Radiation is also often used for pain relief—with or without chemotherapy for inoperable pancreatic cancer—or, for example, for an individual with a painful metastasis to the bone.

Chemotherapy (anticancer agents given by mouth or **intravenously**) is used when you have metastatic disease and in combination with radiation in the postoperative adjuvant setting and for patients with locally advanced disease. The most commonly used drugs are gemcitabine and 5-fluorouracil (5-FU), although several other chemotherapy agents are available. Currently, multiple newer chemotherapy drugs are being studied.

17. What is the difference between curative and palliative treatment?

Curative therapy means trying to get rid of the disease completely and hence hope for a long-term cure. Patients with operable pancreatic cancer have surgery with a curative intent. Nevertheless, because this can-

Adjuvant therapy

use of chemotherapy, radiation therapy, or both following surgical removal of a malignant tumor; used in an attempt to prevent recurrence.

Intravenously

through a vein.

cer may return even after an apparently successful surgery, a true long-term cure is reached in only a few patients. Patients with stage I cancers have the most favorable outcome (approximately 40% will reach the 5-year mark; see Question 14).

Generally, all treatment for inoperable pancreatic cancer (i.e., both locally advanced and metastatic disease) is palliative in nature, which is consistent with the current goals of treatment in advanced pancreatic cancer. In fact, gemcitabine, a relatively newly licensed chemotherapeutic agent for pancreatic cancer, partially achieved approval from the Food and Drug Administration (FDA) based on quality-of-life benefits. Palliative treatment is not useless; relief of symptoms and improving quality of life is a major goal in treating patients with inoperable pancreatic cancer.

18. What is performance status, and how does that influence my treatment choice?

Performance status refers to your ability to function in daily life and generally predicts your tolerance for treatment and overall prognosis. Several medically defined scales (e.g., the Karnofsky scale) can measure your performance status. For example, if you have pancreatic cancer, are receiving treatment, are able to work and function effectively, and have few symptoms from the disease, then you have an excellent performance status. Thus, you are likely to tolerate treatment well, whether it is surgery, chemotherapy, or radiation, and you are also likely to have a better treatment result than someone with cancer who is sickly and who requires help with daily activities (e.g., getting

Relief of symptoms and improving quality of life is a major goal in treating patients with inoperable pancreatic cancer.

Performance status
level of functioning that is scored based on a person's activity during the day and ability to care for him- or herself.

dressed). This latter description refers to a person with a significantly impaired performance status.

Medical **oncologists** (cancer specialists) commonly use performance status scales to help them determine prognosis and to decide on the appropriate treatment. For example, in general, a **clinical trial** (or experimental study) would not be fitting if you have a poor performance status. Gentle chemotherapy or no other treatment besides pain medication might be best for you.

Oncologists

physicians specializing in the treatment of cancer; generally further specialized as medical, surgical, or radiation therapy oncologists.

Clinical trial

research study to test a new treatment on human subjects.

19. What other treatments besides surgery, radiation, and chemotherapy are available?

Several other treatment options are available for patients with pancreatic cancer, one of which would be a clinical trial (see Questions 49 and 50) assessing non-chemotherapy drugs that get in the way of certain cell functions. Several types of vaccines are also being developed as treatments for pancreatic cancer. Some of these vaccines target certain genes in pancreatic cancer and are now beginning to be combined with chemotherapy and radiation in hopes of increasing their effectiveness. Another treatment strategy for pancreatic cancer is a "supportive-care" approach, which means that no active anticancer therapy is employed but that all of the symptom-relieving measures are used (e.g., pain relief, relief of constipation, and drainage of ascites). Supportive-care treatments are included as part of the overall treatment plan for all patients with pancreatic cancer, but in patients with advanced end-stage disease, supportive-care treatments may be used exclusively.

Pain, for some patients with pancreatic cancer, can be a major symptom. Pain-relieving medications are available, although sometimes they are not enough. A **celiac axis** or **nerve block** is a pain-relieving treatment that can be used to control pain and/or cut down on the side effects that some of the pain-relieving medications cause. This route involves putting alcohol and local painkilling agents into the nerve mass that sits behind the pancreas gland. The procedure can be done on an outpatient basis and can be repeated every 8 to 12 weeks if helpful. It is particularly useful if you have back pain and localized pancreatic cancer.

Celiac axis

network of nerves in the upper abdomen.

Nerve block

injection of alcohol or a painkilling medication into a mass of nerves to relieve pain.

Treatment

20. What are the alternative treatments for pancreatic cancer? How do I learn whether these are safe and effective?

Joy's Comment:

Among the "alternative" things that I did was, a year after surgery, I went to see an energy healer in New York; I also saw Dr. Mitchel Gaynor, an oncologist and the author of a book on cancer nutrition, specifically dealing with supplements. He recommended a number of supplements that I took for over a year. I also did yoga (starting about 5 months after surgery), some acupuncture, and had a massage every 3 to 4 weeks. I stopped working and concentrated on spending more time with family and friends, traveling and having fun, and living the most stress-free life that was possible.

Many so-called alternative therapies—that is, those that come from philosophies of health care outside the Western medical mainstream, such as homeopathy or "traditional" medicine—are available for pancreatic

Acupuncture

placement of needles at precise points in the body that are believed to connect with pathways that conduct energy to maintain or restore health.

Always discuss alternative or complementary therapies with your doctor before you use them.

Complementary therapy

a variety of approaches to improve health and treat disease that are not recognized as standard by the traditional medical community but that are used in addition to standard methods of treatment.

Patients can and do survive with good quality of life, sometimes for years.

cancer. Some have legitimate physical benefits (e.g., **acupuncture** as a pain-relieving therapy), others can improve quality of life (e.g., massage and relaxation techniques to reduce stress), but there are some treatments that claim to have medical benefits not substantiated by clinical trials or scientific evidence. Medicines or treatments that are not proven effective through careful research can potentially be dangerous, particularly if you use them in conjunction with other treatments—and *especially* if your doctor does not know you're using them. *Always* discuss alternative or complementary therapies with your doctor before you use them, even if they are something as seemingly harmless as herbal teas—you never know when an ingredient could interact with a chemotherapy or pain medication. You should be especially cautious of treatments that claim to be cures for advanced pancreatic cancer because, unfortunately, the difficult reality of the state of treatment for this disease is that for patients with advanced disease, we speak in terms of prolonging life rather than curing the disease. Conventional treatments simply have not been able to cure advanced pancreatic cancer—yet. Nevertheless, currently available standard treatments do have a useful role. Although pancreatic cancer is difficult to treat, patients can and do survive with good quality of life, sometimes for years—even when diagnosed with advanced disease. Given the limited life expectancy for patients with advanced pancreatic cancer and the limited benefits of standard treatments for patients with advanced pancreatic cancer, it is not surprising that there has been an explosion of non-standard and **complementary therapies** for this disease. Such therapies, when used in conjunction with—*not instead of*—standard therapies, might prove helpful to pancreatic cancer patients. Currently, federal funding is supporting research into some of these treatments to determine the role that they might have, if any, in treating this disease. Pancreatic cancer is a very complex genetic disease, and it is simplistic to think that one approach is going to cure this cancer (other complementary treatments are discussed in Questions 56–58).

21. Why is surgery an option for some people and not others with this cancer?

Joy's Comment:

When I was diagnosed with pancreatic cancer that was operable, I was told that the most important decision in all of my treatment would be to decide on the surgeon. It was recommended that I have the surgery within 2 weeks of the diagnosis. Everyone said Johns Hopkins was the place to go, but I got superb feedback on my surgeon at Stanford Hospital (close to my home). He had done many Whipple surgeries. He's an exceptional surgeon and human being, but I now think the choice of an oncologist who has had lots of pancreatic cancer experience is just as important. If it is impossible to find one nearby, your oncologist should confer with an oncologist with lots of pancreatic cancer experience.

Surgery, for the most part, is appropriate only if the cancer is limited to a small area and if the cancer can be completely removed with no leftover cancer cells at the margin (cut line). For cancers in the head or main portion of the pancreas, a Whipple operation is generally performed. For cancers in the body or tail, partial removal of the pancreas and **spleen** is usually required.

Spleen

an organ in the upper left side of the abdomen that serves to filter the blood.

If you develop jaundice from blockage of the common bile duct and/or develop gastric outlet obstruction (blockage of the opening from the stomach into the

Treatment

27

intestine), an operation can be performed to lessen jaundice and bypass the stomach narrowing. Generally, when both types of blockage are present, a cure is not likely. Nonoperative methods of relieving bile duct and gastric outlet blockages are increasingly being used. An endoscopic plastic or metal stent can be positioned in the common bile duct via an ERCP (endoscopic retrograde cholangiopancreatogram). This latter procedure is somewhat similar to an upper **endoscopy**. Additionally, stents can be placed in the duodenum to relieve gastric outlet blockage, preventing the need for a **surgical bypass**.

If the cancer has metastasized, undergoing surgery usually sets back the time at which you will be able to begin medical treatments (chemotherapy) and offers no real benefit to you. Therefore, as far as possible, it is important that you are examined carefully to decide on the best first step for treatment.

22. What is a Whipple operation, and what side effects should I expect?

A Whipple operation is a major abdominal operation that is performed for cancers that are in the head of the pancreas, the duodenum, or the lower end of the common bile duct. It removes the head of the pancreas, part of the duodenum, and part of the bile duct and also involves reconnecting the bile duct to a different part of the small bowel, connecting a loop of bowel to the stomach, and reconnecting the pancreatic duct to the bowel. At the same time, many lymph nodes are taken out. This is a long-lasting operation that only experienced surgeons should perform.

Endoscopy

procedure for examining the inside of a body tube or of a hollow organ.

Surgical bypass

surgical procedure used when there is a blockage, to create an alternative passage for body substances.

When Whipple operations were first performed several decades ago, the complication and death rates were very high (25% or more). With years of experience, it is now much safer, and in good hands the rate of death is 2% to 3%. However, approximately 30% of the patients still develop problems after the surgery, but most of these are solved without long-term consequences.

Common complications of Whipple surgeries include delayed recovery of stomach movement, resulting in nausea (feeling sick to your stomach or feeling queasy) and vomiting. This side effect can respond to medication and usually goes away with time. Sometimes a surgeon can perform a modified type of Whipple surgery (pylorus sparing procedure) to prevent this from happening. Wound infection and leakage of pancreatic juices are common, but generally get better with simple measures. Diabetes may occur or may be worsened as a result of surgery. Sometimes, the need for glucose-reducing drugs or insulin lessens over time; however, many patients will require treatment for diabetes. Many patients will have lost a large amount of weight before surgery, and most patients will lose approximately 10% to 15% of their total body weight in the 4- to 6-week period after surgery. The reasons for the extreme weight loss are unclear and are unrelated to not eating for an extended period of time. With good dietary advice and nutritional supplements, weight loss can be reduced to some extent. Most patients will never regain a lot of the weight that they lose, and their body weight will remain lower for several months after surgery. Surgery can worsen postoperative weight loss because removal of even part of the pancreas results in loss of digestive enzymes that break down and digest food, which can lead to an inability to absorb important nutrients. Taking supplementary pancreatic enzymes can relieve the side effects that both pancreatic surgery and pancreatic cancer itself cause. Pancreatic enzymes are taken immediately before or during meals on a long-term basis (see Question 61).

John's Comment:

My Whipple surgery took 8 1/2 hours—or so I have been told by my wife! I spent 1 day in the intensive care unit followed by 7 days in the hospital. I had access to intravenous pain medicine throughout my hospital stay, but I only had two or three instances where I used it and only then as a result of muscular pain from twisting my body. I have essentially never had any pain since. During my time in the hospital, I was given a variety of drugs both intravenously and by needle. Some were antibiotics to guard against infection, and one was part of a clinical trial. There were two tubes in my body, one connected to my stomach to relieve pressure and contain nausea and one to my small intestine that served as a feeding tube, through which nutrients were pumped into my body. These tubes remained for about 3 months; I didn't take anything approaching solid food for more than a week, and it was a good 4 months before my digestive system functioned as it should and as it does now.

23. What other types of operations are used for pancreatic cancer?

The location of the cancer in the pancreas determines the type of operation. Pancreatic adenocarcinomas can be in the head and neck of the gland, in which case a Whipple operation is performed. For tumors in the body, several types of operations can be performed, including Whipple surgery, removal of the mid portion of the pancreas alone, or a distal pancreatectomy, in which the surgeon removes the mid and tail portions of the pancreas and the spleen (because of blood vessel supply) and sometimes part of your stomach.

24. I have just undergone a Whipple surgery for pancreatic cancer and was told that all of my disease was removed. Am I cured?

Whipple surgeries are performed in patients with pancreatic cancer with an intent to cure. The best outcome is when all of the disease is removed. This occurs in many patients; however, for most, cancer does return in the future. We do not understand why pancreatic cancer returns after an apparently successful surgery, but we assume that it is related to the biology of the cancer. The best outcome from surgery is found when you have a small (less than 2 cm) cancer with no lymph nodes involved and no remaining cancer cells at the cut line. In these circumstances, that is, a stage I cancer, approximately 40% of patients will live for 5 years; however, for many of the patients that have surgery, lymph node involvement is identified, signifying a prognosis that is not as good. On average, after surgery, survival is expected to be between approximately 13 and 20 months, and on average, the cancer returns at approximately 1 year. These figures are statistical averages and do not refer to individual patients. Several large databases of patients who have undergone surgery for pancreatic cancer have shown that the cancer comes back in most of the patients at some point, sometimes as late as 5 years after the surgery. If the cancer returns, it is considered treatable, but the long-term prognosis is worse in patients who have returning pancreatic cancer.

Thus, in all likelihood, a Whipple surgery may not be a true long-term cure for pancreatic cancer; however, it is the best available tool if the cancer is limited to a small area. Hence, if surgery is possible, you should undergo attempted removal of the cancer. Adjuvant therapy (or postoperative chemotherapy and radiation or chemotherapy alone) after surgery may be considered to reduce the chance that the cancer will return. Adjuvant therapy is controversial and is discussed more thoroughly in Question 41.

Whipple surgery may not be a true long-term cure for pancreatic cancer; however, it is the best available tool.

Joy's Comment:

Two years after my Whipple surgery, I had recurrence—a small tumor on the left iliac bone and 2 small tumors around the rectal area. This location is extremely rare for pancreatic cancer recurrence. I again had radiation and 5-FU (in the pill form, Xeloda).

25. My doctor says that my cancer is localized but that they can't operate. Why?

The major reason that apparently localized pancreatic cancer might be considered inoperable is that the cancer is surrounding some major blood vessels that cannot be removed. Certain blood vessels, including the superior mesenteric artery, the celiac axis, the portal vein, the hepatic artery, and sometimes the superior mesenteric vein, simply cannot be operated upon without a very serious risk to the patient, although in expert surgical hands part of the portal vein can occasionally be taken out and rebuilt. An experimental option is artery grafting; however, this approach has not been proven sound and is usually not a practical and safe option. If the blood vessels cannot be removed, a complete microscopic removal of the cancer is not possible, and hence the patient is unlikely to benefit from the operation. Surgery should always remove all evidence (however small it may be) of the cancer; otherwise, the patient is subjected to the problems of a major operation without the benefits of long-term control of the cancer.

26. If the cancer has spread outside of the pancreas, is surgery ever a possibility?

Yes. The major reasons for surgery are to manage jaundice from blockage of the common bile duct or to relieve a blockage of the outlet from the stomach (gastric outlet obstruction). If both of these complications are present together, then surgery deals best with these problems. If blockage of the bile duct occurs on its own, placing an endoscopic plastic or metal wall stent (like a piece of piping) with an ERCP procedure serves the patient better. If gastric outlet blockage is present on its own, a similar type of metal stent can be put in the duodenum to wedge open the small bowel and to allow the patient to eat and drink.

Nevertheless, every attempt to avoid surgery is generally made if the cancer has spread because the surgical recovery period may be long and will not increase a patient's overall life expectancy.

27. If I can't have surgery, do I still have a chance of being cured?

In general, cure is not possible if surgery cannot be performed. There are individual reports of long-term survivors with pancreatic adenocarcinoma who have undergone combined chemotherapy and radiation for locally advanced (inoperable, but not spread) pancreatic cancer. Such individuals are not considered to be the norm of what happens in advanced pancreatic cancer... but they *do* exist. The most realistic assessment of such cases is that they are extremely unusual.

28. What happens if my disease comes back? How is a return diagnosed and treated? Is it possible to stay alive if the pancreatic cancer returns?

A return of pancreatic adenocarcinoma following successful surgery is common and is the rule rather than the exception. Most recurrences are seen within a year of surgery and are identified in many different ways. Sometimes regular CT scans identify new evidence of metastatic disease (e.g., involving the liver or peritoneum). Patients often develop symptoms (fatigue, weight loss, decreased appetite, or pain) indicating a return of cancer. Any new and constant symptoms in a patient with pancreatic cancer who has undergone surgery should be investigated. Occasionally, a recurrence may be suspected but is difficult to prove. When this happens, serial monitoring with CT scans or an MRI and physical assessment of the patient will allow the diagnosis to be proven or disproven. **Tumor markers** or blood tests that identify substances secreted by the cancer (e.g., Ca19–9 or carcinoembryonic antigen

Any new and constant symptoms in a patient with pancreatic cancer who has undergone surgery should be investigated.

Tumor markers

substances produced by malignant tumors that can be measured in the blood.

[CEA]) can be measured, and a progressive rise in the number values of these markers may predict the return of cancer. The rise in markers will often be apparent several months before symptoms are present or before solid evidence is shown on a scan; however, using tumor markers as the only way to determine a recurrence is not recommended. In fact, many experts suggest that tumor markers should not be used at all because they may cause you to worry and do not change the long-term result.

Joy's Comment:

My Ca19–9 started to rise a year after my Whipple surgery. My doctors monitored it and eventually stated that there was probably some tumor activity, but because I felt good and nothing showed on the CT scan, they recommended no treatment. About 9 months after the beginning of the rise in Ca19–9, I began to feel some pain around my rectal area. The doctors dismissed this as being related to pancreatic cancer because (1) they had never seen pancreatic cancer recur in that area and (2) nothing showed on the scan. However, about 4 months later, an MRI and PET scan showed tumors on the left iliac bone and by the rectum, and I began another treatment of radiation and chemotherapy, followed by a continuing program of combined chemotherapy drugs, and the tumor marker is currently falling.

29. What is chemotherapy?

Chemotherapy is medical drug treatment that is usually given intravenously (but occasionally by mouth) to treat cancers. Chemotherapy drugs are also called cytotoxic drugs, which means they are cell-destroying medications. Many different types of chemotherapeutic drugs exist that affect cancer cells in different ways by altering or interfering with differing parts of the cell cycle. Sometimes chemotherapy drugs are given alone and sometimes in a combination to try and achieve better control of the cancer.

Chemotherapy drugs affect rapidly dividing cells in the body, including cancer cells. The reason that side effects occur from chemotherapy is partly related to these effects on the more rapidly turning over cells, (e.g., hair loss or irritation of the lining of the mouth or the lining of the bowel [diarrhea]). In addition, some chemotherapy drugs have other side effects that are specific to that drug or class of drugs. Side effects of chemotherapy are also related to the dose and frequency of administration of the drugs as well as to characteristics of the patient (e.g., healthy, strong patients tolerate chemotherapy much better than sick, debilitated patients). Medication is sometimes required to minimize or counteract the side effects of chemotherapy.

30. What chemotherapy drugs are used to treat pancreatic cancer? What are the FDA-licensed treatments for pancreatic cancer?

Many different chemotherapeutic agents (some well-established and some new) are used to treat pancreatic cancer. Traditionally, 5-FU was used most often to treat pancreatic cancer; however, for the most part, gemcitabine (Gemzar) has replaced it for patients with inoperable pancreatic cancer. Some of the other drugs that are used to treat pancreatic adenocarcinoma include irinotecan (CPT–11, Camptosar), docetaxel

(Taxotere), cisplatin, mitomycin, and paclitaxel (Taxol).

For metastatic pancreatic cancer, gemcitabine is the main drug used and is usually given intravenously over 30 minutes weekly for 3 of 4 weeks. Gemcitabine is a fairly well-tolerated chemotherapy agent, with the main side effects including some nausea, fatigue, low blood counts, flu-like symptoms, and rarely hair thinning. Gemcitabine on its own has been shown to be better than 5-FU in treating inoperable pancreatic cancer in terms of both quality-of-life benefits (decreased pain, improved well-being, etc.) and duration of life. Gemcitabine is increasingly being combined with other drugs such as irinotecan, docetaxel, and cisplatin as a method of increasing control of the cancer. Giving gemcitabine over a longer period of time (i.e., over 90 minutes instead of the more usual 30-minute schedule) may be beneficial, although we are unsure whether this way of delivering drugs is better. Two downsides to giving gemcitabine over a longer period of time are an increase in flu-like symptoms and a drop in the blood counts. For now, lengthened delivery of gemcitabine remains an experimental option.

Gemcitabine, 5-FU, and mitomycin are the FDA-licensed drugs for treating pancreatic cancer. FDA licensure of a drug means that it has been specifically evaluated for use in treating a specific disease (in this case, pancreatic cancer) and compared with the best available therapies at that time for the disease. Many other drugs for pancreatic cancer, as noted previously, although not FDA-licensed for treatment of pancreatic cancer, have also been thoroughly reviewed. Thus, to some extent, FDA licensure does not truly determine common clinical practice. The last drug to be FDA licensed for pancreatic adenocarcinoma was gemcitabine in June 1996. Several other drugs for pancreatic adenocarcinoma in the late stages (Phase III) of clinical trial assessment may come up for licensure in the coming 1 to 2 years.

31. Are two or more chemotherapy drugs given together better than just one when treating pancreatic cancer?

As of 2002, it is unclear whether a two-drug gemcitabine-based combination for treating patients with metastatic pancreatic adenocarcinoma is better than gemcitabine alone. The rising two-drug combinations are gemcitabine combined with cisplatin, irinotecan, docetaxel, or an experimental drug called DX–8951f, which is related to irinotecan. The advantages of a two-drug combination are as follows: a greater short-term ability to shrink the cancer and the possibility of relieving symptoms more quickly. The disadvantages of multiple drug combinations are the greater potential for side effects, including lower **white blood cell** and **platelet** counts (predisposing to infection and bleeding, respectively), as well as more tiredness, hair loss, and nausea, among other side effects. Multiple clinical trials are underway in the United States, Canada, and Europe to see whether two-drug gemcitabine-based combinations are better than gemcitabine alone. The results of some of these studies will be available in 1 to 2 years. We think that for patients with a good performance status (i.e., someone who is reasonably strong), two-drug combinations may be superior to gemcitabine alone.

White blood cells

a variety of blood cells that fight infection.

Platelet

blood cells that stop bleeding by clumping together to plug a damaged blood vessel.

Joy's Comment:

My current oncologist, who has many pancreatic cancer patients, believes strongly in combinations of drugs. I am currently on a combination of Gemzar and Taxotere; before this I was on Xeloda and mitomycin.

32. What are the expected benefits from chemotherapy in pancreatic cancer?

Chemotherapy in pancreatic cancer is given to (1) control the cancer, (2) improve the quality of life, and (3) increase the length of life. Because pancreatic cancer that has spread is not curable, quality-of-life issues are important when considering chemotherapy.

Quality-of-life issues are important when considering chemotherapy.

To date, gemcitabine is the most effective single drug in treating advanced pancreatic cancer. The trials that have been carried out show that on average a patient with advanced pancreatic cancer will have a short-term shrinkage of his or her disease approximately 10% of the time, will have an average life expectancy of about 5.5 months, and will have an approximately 18% chance of living to 1 year. These figures are statistical averages and do not refer to individual patients, and some patients will have smaller volumes of cancer and would be expected to fare better than these statistics suggest.

Gemcitabine received FDA licensure in 1996 partly because of improved quality-of-life benefits. The first trials were conducted in patients who had pain from pancreatic adenocarcinoma. In approximately 25% of patients who received gemcitabine, pain levels were reduced, and a lesser amount of pain medication was needed. In addition, these patients tended to live somewhat longer than patients who received the comparator drug, 5-FU. In a smaller number of patients,

39

improvement in dry weight (i.e., not fluid gain) was also observed. In contrast, only about 5% of patients who received 5-FU had any quality-of-life benefit from the chemotherapy.

Joy's Comment:

I was much sicker from radiation (and from the first day) than from chemotherapy, but each drug is different (the most noticeable difference was a lack of energy, but not consistently). Occasionally, on Gemzar, I had chills and fever. Lack of appetite is always an issue for me when on chemotherapy, and nausea was an issue from radiation. I took Kytril, which helped but made me constipated, so I stopped taking it. Mostly I just ate "soft" foods, drank Boost, and lost weight!

33. What are the side effects from chemotherapy?

Chemotherapy side effects can be divided into general chemotherapy side effects and drug-specific side effects. To some extent, almost everybody has some side effects from chemotherapy. In most patients, side effects are tolerable and treatable; in a few, however, chemotherapy side effects can be significant and occasionally life threatening. In advanced pancreatic cancer, making the chemotherapy treatment as easy to manage as possible is a major goal. Gemcitabine, for the most part, fulfills this requirement.

In most patients, side effects are tolerable and treatable.

General side effects of chemotherapy include nausea, tiredness, a sense of ill-being, hair thinning, and a drop in blood counts. A drop in white blood cells, which fight infection in your body, puts you at risk for infection. For gemcitabine, the degree of drop in the white cell count is usually fairly small and does not last long (2 to 3 days), making the risk for infection quite low.

The platelets (clotting factors in the blood) may also drop because of chemotherapy. Again, for gemcitabine, this drop is brief and is usually not of clinical importance. Bleeding has rarely been seen as a complication of this drug when given on its own.

More specific side effects of chemotherapy relate to the drug or class to which the drug belongs. For gemcitabine, these side effects include flu-like symptoms (fevers, aches, and tiredness) that usually last for 2 to 3 days after chemotherapy. Other side effects of gemcitabine can include ankle swelling, skin rashes, a brief rise of liver blood tests, and rarely kidney problems.

John's Comment:

I was very fortunate. Other than losses of energy and some weight, I experienced no side effects from radiotherapy and chemotherapy. M. D. Anderson, the cancer center where I was treated, administered an antinausea drug with the chemotherapy and radiation (in my case, gemcitabine was the chemotherapy agent), and it is very effective. The loss of energy and strength was significant—there were days when I just lay around in the sun all day. With the wonderful and necessary assistance of my primary care person, my wife, I was able to commute from California to Houston for my last three chemotherapy sessions.

34. What is radiation therapy?

Radiation therapy is x-ray treatment used to control and cure different types of cancer. Radiation is like surgery in that it is a localized type of treatment that affects small areas in the body, and it is different from chemotherapy, which circulates throughout the body. Radiation treatment is usually delivered daily, Monday to Friday. A treatment course, depending on the area being treated and on the size of the cancer, can be any-where from 5–10 treatments to 28–35 treatments. Very specific targets are marked out on your body, often using complicated CT scanning to determine the exact area to be treated. This process (called **simulation**) can take several hours. From there, medical physicists and the radiation oncologist plan the total dose of the radi-ation, the number of treatments, and the field size. Usually a couple of days before beginning radiation, you will undergo a "beam check" to ensure that the radiation prescription is exact and appropriate. Each daily radiation treatment takes approximately 10 min-utes.

Simulation

procedure that is part of the planning process for the administration of radiation therapy; involves x-rays or CT scans to identify the area to be treated and tattooing the skin to ensure correct positioning each day of treatment.

For pancreatic cancer, radiation treatment planning can be challenging because of the nearness of the stomach, the small bowel, the spinal cord, etc. Gener-ally, after a treatment course has been administered, no further radiation can be delivered to that specific area because of effects to other normal surrounding organs and structures.

35. What is combined modality therapy (chemoradiation)?

Combined modality therapy or chemoradiation refers to the simultaneous delivery of chemotherapy and radiation. It is often used in the postoperative adjuvant setting and for patients with locally advanced inopera-ble pancreatic cancer.

There is a good reason for administering chemother-apy and radiation at the same time. Chemotherapy acts as a radiation sensitizer or potentiator, making radiation more effective in controlling the tumor in the irradiated field. The most commonly used chemotherapy drug with radiation is 5-FU, which can be given as an injection for 3 to 5 days during the first week and also during the 5th week of concurrent treatment. One other commonly used method of administering 5-FU with radiation is to deliver the 5-FU as a continuous intravenous infusion. This means that you would wear a little pump, like a baby's bottle, around your waist, and the 5-FU flows continuously into a central vein via a **mediport**. The 5-FU is delivered in this way throughout the full 5- to 6-week course of radiation, if you do not have excessive side effects from it. Gemcitabine is increasingly being used as a radiation sensitizer; however, the best way to give gemcitabine combined with radiation has not been defined. In addition, the combination of the two may cause significant side effects and for now is best used in a carefully monitored clinical trial. One of the other qualities of chemotherapy when given with radiation is that it can go around the body and can theoretically deal with any small cells that may have escaped.

36. What other types of radiation are used to treat pancreatic cancer? What is intraoperative radiation therapy? What is stereotactic radiation?

External beam radiation therapy (radiation administered from outside the body) is typically used to treat pancreatic cancer in the postoperative adjuvant setting and also to treat patients with locally advanced pancreatic cancer.

Intraoperative radiation therapy (IORT) is given during surgery because a high dose of radiation can be directed to the cancer itself, minimizing the effects on

Treatment

Mediport

device implanted under the skin with a connecting catheter that is threaded into a large vein in the chest; provides a way to draw blood and administer chemotherapy.

External beam radiation therapy

radiation therapy administered by a machine in which a beam of radiation is directed to a defined part of the body.

Intraoperative radiation therapy

administration of radiation therapy at the time of surgery.

normal surrounding tissues. Multiple studies have looked at the value of giving radiation this way and have demonstrated that control of the cancer in the pancreatic area is better with this treatment (i.e., the local recurrence rate is reduced); however, no clear-cut influence on overall survival or length of life has been identified as a result of IORT. IORT requires a high level of skill and a specially designed operating room and is not routinely performed for pancreatic cancer.

Stereotactic radiation is another strategy for delivering external beam radiation (as opposed to IORT). It involves a very localized administration of high-dose radiation to the pancreas cancer and has also been used to treat liver metastases from pancreatic cancer. In some patients, stereotactic radiation may help to treat pancreatic cancer; however, it currently does not have a defined role.

Stereotactic radiation

administration of radiation therapy using special devices to pinpoint the beam of radiation to a small precisely defined region.

37. What are the expected benefits of radiation in pancreatic cancer?

Radiation is generally given in three situations for the treatment of pancreatic cancer: (1) as a definitive treatment for locally advanced, inoperable pancreatic cancer; (2) as postoperative adjuvant therapy to reduce the return of pancreatic cancer after surgery; or (3) as a method of pain relief. When used for definitive or adjuvant treatment, radiation is typically administered over a 5- to 6-week period. In these cases, chemotherapy is usually used concurrently with radiation. When used for pain relief, radiation is used alone, and it typically is administered over 10–15 days.

Radiation on its own does not have the ability to cure pancreatic cancer, most likely because of early spread of disease to other parts of the body at a microscopic level.

38. What are the side effects of radiation?

The side effects of radiation depend on what part of your body is being irradiated. For most patients with pancreatic cancer, the radiation field will be the pancreas itself; however, radiation will occasionally be used at a site of bony cancer spread for pain control. The side effects of irradiating your pancreas depend on what happens to the normal nearby tissues. Principally, nausea and irritation of the lining of the stomach are common, especially toward the end of a course of radiation. Fatigue or tiredness is also a well-recognized side effect of treatment. Other side effects include lowering of white blood cell and platelet counts (see Questions 68 and 69), which is generally short-term and may result in a brief break from the radiation delivery. You may see some long-lasting (but usually mild) darkening of the skin and skin dryness in the mid back area (Question 63), which often fades over time. Skin burns rarely occur with radiation. Radiation to the pancreas, along with surgery and pancreatic cancer itself, may increase the likelihood of developing pancreatic insufficiency or malabsorption from decreased production of pancreatic enzymes. However, pancreatic enzymes can be taken before meals, particularly with meals containing high fat, to offset this problem (see Question 61).

Radiation on its own does not have the ability to cure pancreatic cancer.

Treatment

39. What is adjuvant therapy and what is neoadjuvant therapy?

Adjuvant therapy is treatment given after surgery to lessen your chances that the cancer will return. Neoadjuvant therapy is the same type of treatment, except that it is given before surgery.

A strong historical precedent for adjuvant therapy for pancreatic cancer dates back to the late 1970s and early 1980s. Traditionally, adjuvant therapy involves a combination of chemotherapy and radiation. Increasingly, chemotherapy is being used alone. New treatment strategies such as vaccination approaches and new biologic agents (or non–chemotherapy-type agents) are also being assessed in the postoperative adjuvant setting.

Neoadjuvant therapy or preoperative chemoradiation is an appealing strategy for several reasons. First, it offers definitive treatment of the cancer by selecting out patients who are destined to develop metastatic disease early (occurs in about 20% to 25% of patients) and are therefore spared a surgery that was going to be of no benefit to them anyway. Second, chemotherapy and radiation may be somewhat more effective when given preoperatively because for maximum effect, radiation requires well-oxygenated tissues, which are present before surgery upsets the blood supply. Third, it is possible that preoperative chemoradiation may make a few borderline patients operable. It is important to stress that the latter theoretic benefit is realized in a tiny portion of patients with nonoperable pancreatic adenocarcinoma. Fourth, the ability to deliver preoperative therapy is higher compared with postoperative chemoradiation, where greater than 25% of possible patients are unable to receive treatment because of delayed postoperative recovery or other problems. Some of the major medical institutions in the United States frequently recommend preoperative chemoradiation, whereas in most other parts of the world and in many centers in the United States, it would not be offered as a standard option. Currently, no definitive studies are available that compare preoperative with postoperative therapy to help decide which might be the better approach. For now, preoperative chemoradiation is an investigational and not a standard option.

40. What are the specific adjuvant therapies that may be recommended to me?

Traditional adjuvant therapy involves a combination of chemotherapy and radiation, usually beginning within 4 to 6 weeks after surgery. Radiation therapy is delivered over approximately 28 days—that is, each working day (Monday through Friday) for almost six weeks. Chemotherapy is administered by various methods at the same time as radiation. One option is to give the chemotherapeutic agent 5-FU on the first 3 to 5 and last 3 to 5 days of radiation. Another approach is to give a continuous infusion of 5-FU throughout the radiation period via a small "pump" that you wear around your waist. Gemcitabine is increasingly being given at the same time as radiation in the postoperative adjuvant setting; however, this is currently not considered to be a standard of care.

After combined chemotherapy and radiation are completed, further weekly chemotherapy for a several-month period is an option, but the additional benefits that this may offer are unclear.

In Europe, following a large clinical trial (the European Study Group for Pancreatic Cancer's first study, also referred to as ESPAC–1), enthusiasm for giving chemotherapy and radiation together after surgery has declined. In Europe, chemotherapy alone is increasingly being used as a postoperative therapy, usually with 5-FU and occasionally with gemcitabine. Some disagreement among pancreatic cancer experts exists about this approach, although these differences may reflect styles of practice rather than actual differences in outcome.

41. How effective is adjuvant therapy?

Adjuvant therapy is a controversial postoperative treatment for patients who have had complete resection of pancreatic cancer. When the first clinical trials that explored adjuvant therapy for pancreas cancer were conducted in the 1970s and early 1980s, a clear-cut positive benefit for adjuvant therapy was identified; however, the trials included very small numbers of patients, limiting the statistical conclusions. The treatment design for the chemoradiation is considered old by current standards, and also Whipple surgery has become a much safer operation over the past two decades, lessening the apparent differences between surgery alone and surgery and chemoradiation. We note that currently, a national trial of adjuvant therapy in pancreatic cancer—only the second one ever conducted—is underway and nearing completion, so standards may change as the results of this trial become known.

In Europe, as noted in Question 40, the approach to adjuvant therapy is different, with the major emphasis being on chemotherapy alone and not on radiation. In fact, the current ongoing major European trial (ESPAC–3) does not contain radiation at all as part of the adjuvant treatment. In addition, many experts worldwide feel that adjuvant therapy has never been adequately shown to influence the long-term outcome of pancreatic cancer. We believe that a few patients likely benefit from adjuvant therapy and that this group has a better prognosis to start (e.g., small cancer with no lymph nodes involved), but in reality, adjuvant therapy of any type at this time, although offered to a majority of patients, probably benefits few. You should discuss and decide on the best plan with your doctor. The disagreements over the benefits of adjuvant therapy make obvious another point: *there is a pressing need to develop better therapies for this disease.*

42. Are there any experimental programs for people who have undergone apparently successful surgery to try and prevent the cancer from returning?

A number of experimental treatments are being assessed in the postoperative (adjuvant) setting for patients who have had complete removal of a pancreatic cancer. Some of these include vaccine programs, and some involve the use of new biologic (non–chemotherapeutic-type) agents. One vaccine approach has been to immunize patients against an abnormal gene (the *ras* gene), or piece of DNA, that is unique to pancreatic cancer cells. Early results show that the approach appears to be very safe and well tolerated; however, it remains to be seen what influence, if any, vaccine strategies have on the overall outcomes in pancreatic cancer.

43. What are the specific treatment options for locally advanced pancreatic cancer?

Treatment options for locally advanced pancreatic cancer include (1) combined chemotherapy and radiation, (2) chemotherapy alone, (3) clinical trials, and (4) supportive care alone. The traditional treatment for locally advanced disease is combined **chemoradiotherapy**. However, chemotherapy alone is the emerging treatment based on the high rate of spread of this cancer to other areas of the body. For any stage of pancreatic cancer, clinical trials are an important therapeutic consideration. For the combined chemoradiotherapy option, the typical radiosensitizer is 5-FU, but again, like in other areas of treatment of disease with chemoradiotherapy, gemcitabine is becoming the radiosensitizer. For patients receiving chemotherapy alone, gemcitabine or a gemcitabine-based combination is the mainstay of therapy. If you are not well enough for active treatment, a supportive or symptom-relieving approach is used. Where there is a choice of treatment options, from the available data using currently available drugs and modern radiotherapeutic principles, superiority of chemoradiation over chemotherapy alone has not been demonstrated. The decision is for you and your physician to make.

Chemoradio-therapy

combined modality therapy, treatment with a combination of chemotherapy and radiation therapy.

Clinical trials are an important therapeutic consideration.

44. What are the specific treatment options for metastatic pancreatic cancer?

For metastatic pancreatic cancer, the backbone of treatment is chemotherapy. Surgery rarely has a role, except in relief of gastric outlet blockage and possibly for relief of jaundice caused by blockage of the com-

For metastatic pancreatic cancer, the backbone of treatment is chemotherapy.

mon bile duct. The chemotherapy options include (1) gemcitabine alone, (2) gemcitabine-based two-drug combinations, (3) clinical trials, and (4) supportive care. For those who are weakened because of disease, the main options include either gemcitabine on its own or a supportive-care approach. For strong individuals with advanced pancreatic cancer, the emphasis should be on new treatments or clinical trials or possibly gemcitabine-based chemotherapy combinations. To date, no clearly better option over single-agent gemcitabine has appeared. However, several studies are underway that look at some of the newer agents and compare them with the standard therapy (gemcitabine). It is likely that results about some of these new drugs will be available over the coming 1 to 2 years.

If at all possible, a medical oncology opinion at a major academic institution with an interest in pancreatic cancer can help you to lay out the most suitable and useful treatment options. If possible, this consultation should be done before beginning specific treatment.

45. How do I know whether my treatment is working?

Your physician's clinical assessment, blood tests, and CT results are the key methods of finding out whether your pancreatic cancer treatment is helpful. If you have symptoms from cancer (e.g., pain, weight loss, and decreased appetite), you may notice that chemotherapy improves some of these. Such an observation, although subjective, would suggest that treatment is indeed beneficial. More concrete methods of cancer assessment include a direct comparison of radiologic imaging (e.g., CT scans or MRI) before and after a given treatment. In general, if a chemotherapy treatment for metastatic pancreatic cancer is resulting in either unchanged or improved radiologic findings and acceptable treatment-related side effects, then treatment is assumed to be beneficial. In contrast, if there is definite growth of the cancer or worsening of quality of life because of treatment-related problems, then the entire risk–benefit equation needs to be evaluated again, which would generally result in a change of treatment.

You may wonder about how long the therapy should continue if treatment is helping (i.e., the cancer is stable or improved). Again, there is no clear-cut right answer here, and you and your physician should make this decision. We think that if you are tolerating treatment well and are not developing increasing treatment-related side effects and have stable or improved disease, then treatment should probably continue for 6 to 12 months. However, there is uncertainty in the field about this opinion.

Tumor markers or blood tests (e.g., CEA and Ca19–9) can be done periodically to assess response. Tumor markers are substances secreted into the blood stream by tumor cells; however, they are currently not a dependable method for determining benefit from a particular treatment, as the levels can vary for reasons other than growth or shrinkage of the cancer. Many clinical trials use a tumor marker measurement at regular intervals to assess further whether the degree of rise or the rate of change of a tumor marker may predict growth of the cancer.

John's Comment:

I return to M. D. Anderson for a checkup every 6 months. Initially I returned every 3 months, but that was lengthened after my 1-year anniversary. I fly into Houston on Sunday night and have blood drawn that evening. The next day, I have a chest x-ray and a CT scan with contrast. On Day 2, I meet with my surgeon to review the results of the tests and then fly back to California that day.

46. What does a "complete response" mean? What does a "partial response" mean? What are the implications of a complete response or partial response?

A **complete response** describes when someone with cancer has a complete disappearance of all radiologic disease and an end of all cancer-related symptoms as a result of treatment. It is used to measure the benefit of treatment from chemotherapeutic agents generally in the context of a clinical trial. For patients with pancreatic cancer who are receiving the best currently available chemotherapies, complete responses are very rare. They are seen more commonly in chemotherapy-sensitive cancers such as breast or ovarian cancer.

A **partial response** refers to a large decrease in the volume of cancer as measured radiographically (an improvement of 50% or better) without the growth of any new tumors in the body. Partial responses often occur with currently available chemotherapeutic agents. For example, the partial response rate is approximately 10% to 12% with gemcitabine alone in metastatic pancreatic cancer. This means that 10 to 12 patients of 100 treated will have some solid evidence of

Complete response

disappearance of all signs of disease as a result of treatment.

Partial response

decrease in the size of a tumor, by at least 50%, as a result of treatment.

temporary tumor reduction. The complete response rate to gemcitabine alone is almost 0%. In contrast, for gemcitabine-based drug combinations, a partial response rate of 20% to 30% or more might be anticipated. This does not necessarily imply that the treatment is better, and in addition, there may be more side effects from more drugs.

Partial responses, or more rarely complete responses, in pancreatic cancer are often short lived, usually for a period of weeks to several months; however, sometimes long-lasting control of pancreatic cancer for a year or more can be obtained from chemotherapy treatments.

47. What does "stable disease" mean? What are the implications of stable disease?

Stable disease

no growth of a tumor; considered a favorable situation for patients with pancreatic cancer.

Stable disease is when there is no significant growth in a patient's cancer on a given therapy. Stable disease, if the treatment is tolerated acceptably, is a positive situation in pancreatic adenocarcinoma. Generally, a stable disease state would prompt continuation of the current therapy.

48. What is progression of disease? What happens if my tumor continues growing during treatment?

Progression

growth of a tumor or spread of a tumor to a distant site in the body.

Progression of disease describes clear-cut growth or spread of your cancer. The term can be used in either a clinical sense (e.g., your pain is worse or you are continuing to lose weight) or a radiologic sense, where a comparison of before and after scans shows growth of the cancer. Progression of cancer demands a change in the treatment plan. Sometimes this might mean switching chemotherapy treatment or participation in a clinical trial, or for some who are very weakened by their cancer, it may mean stopping active treatment and beginning a supportive care approach.

Pancreatic cancer is resistant to chemotherapy, and thus, progression is commonly seen. Your treating oncologist should advise you on the next steps. Keep in mind the extent of your prior treatment and your level of well-being and laboratory issues, etc.

Progression of cancer demands a change in the treatment plan.

49. What is a clinical trial?

Clinical trials are research studies that are designed to test new treatments on humans, including drugs (chemotherapy), methods of administering radiation therapy, immunologic agents, nutritional therapies, medical devices, or even behavioral therapies. A single new treatment or standard treatments combined in new ways may be studied. Therapeutic clinical trials can be divided into Phases I, II, III, and IV. Most pancreatic oncology trials are therapeutic trials, as opposed to screening or prevention trials, and are concerned with Phases I–III.

Participating in a clinical trial is not being a "guinea pig." These studies are designed thoughtfully, building on information that we have previously learned about the new treatment. To protect your safety, the FDA strictly controls and watches how clinical trials are conducted. The study must undergo review at the hospital with which the doctor is associated and must be approved and monitored by an institutional review board. In addition, each study has specific eligibility

Participating in a clinical trial is not being a "guinea pig."

Treatment

criteria describing precisely who can be treated in the study. A further step to protect people enrolled in clinical trials is that everyone receives a consent form describing the purpose of the study, the treatment that they will receive, the possible side effects of treatment, the risks and benefits, and the financial costs of treatment. Before receiving any treatment, you must sign this consent form indicating that you understand the study and that you agree to participate. The key things that you need to understand before enrolling in a clinical trial are (1) the purpose of the study, (2) the possible risks and benefits to you, (3) the duration of the study, (4) the tests involved, and (5) the cost to you and your insurance carrier.

Participating in a clinical trial offers you the opportunity to receive new treatments before they are available to others. You receive care by a leading doctor who is associated with a major cancer center, and you are closely monitored throughout your treatment. You are also able to contribute to progress in medical science. It is important, however, to remember that the treatment given in a clinical trial is not yet proven to be more effective than the standard treatment that you might receive, and there may even be side effects that were not expected. Furthermore, you may have to spend more time receiving treatment, having special diagnostic tests, and seeing the doctor. In addition, there may be more financial costs to you. Some aspects of care may not be covered by your health insurance, and you may have costs of transportation or housing if the treatment is not close to home. There is no right thing to do; the decision as to whether to participate in a clinical trial is ultimately yours (see Question 51 for information on how to find a clinical trial).

50. What are Phase I, II, and III clinical trials?

New treatments are usually first developed in a laboratory and are then tested in animals. If they seem to offer something promising, they are tested in phases in humans to determine their safety and effectiveness.

A Phase I clinical trial is an early clinical trial that looks at new drugs or combinations of established drugs. The most important goals of a Phase I study are to determine the dose, side effects, and schedule for giving the treatment. Phase I studies are usually not restricted to a specific type of cancer; therefore, patients with a varied range of cancers might be qualified for a given Phase I study. Phase I studies usually include relatively small group of patients (often 14 to 50) and are often done at just one institution.

A Phase II clinical trial expands on information obtained in a Phase I study. Generally, a new drug is assessed in a specific disease and often a specific stage of disease. The major goal of a Phase II study is to determine how effective the treatment is. Additional information is gathered on safety and tolerability. Phase II clinical trials are usually fairly small (20 to 50 patients).

A Phase III clinical trial is generally a comparison of the new therapy against the current standard treatment for a particular type of cancer. Patients are randomly assigned to receive either the standard treatment or the new treatment. You cannot select which treatment you want to get. Phase III trials are often large—several hundred patients—and are often conducted at multiple institutions and sometimes multiple countries and multiple continents. They may take several years to complete. If an experimental treatment is demonstrated to be superior to a standard therapy in a Phase III trial, if the trial is well-conducted and scientifically valid, and if the new treatment is adequately tolerated, the experimental drug may get FDA approval for that disease.

51. How can I find a clinical trial for pancreatic cancer that would be right for me?

If you are interested in participating in a clinical trial, you should ask your doctor for a recommendation.

If you are interested in participating in a clinical trial, you should ask your doctor for a recommendation. It may be better to hold off starting treatment until you have looked into the options and until you have discussed with your doctor whether this is appropriate. Also, because of the eligibility criteria for each clinical trial, you should know the type and stage of pancreatic cancer that you have: resectable, locally advanced, or metastatic. Your doctor can give you this information.

You may want to ask your doctor to find the clinical trials that are available. You could also call a National Cancer Institute-designated comprehensive cancer center in your region and speak with a research nurse, who can inform you of the available clinical trials. A number of organizations provide listings of clinical trials for pancreatic cancer:

- Pancreatic Cancer Action Network (*www.pancan. org* or 1–877–2-PANCAN)
- Pancreatica (*www.pancreatica.org*)
- National Cancer Institute (*www.cancer.gov/ clinical_trials* or 1–800–4-CANCER; their publication, *Taking Part in Clinical Trials: What Cancer Patients Need to Know*, is an excellent resource and is available from the Cancer Information Service of the National Cancer Institute)
- National Institutes of Health (*www.clinicaltrials.gov*)
- Coalition of National Cancer Cooperative Groups (*www.cancertrialshelp.org* or 1–877–520–4457)
- Centerwatch, an information services company, which provides a listing of clinical trials (*www.centerwatch.com*).

52. What new drugs are being assessed in pancreatic cancer?

As the currently available treatments for pancreatic cancer often have little or no impact on many patients, new drugs are constantly being assessed. These new drugs can be classified under new chemotherapeutic (cytotoxic) agents, new biologic agents, or new other strategies. Most of these agents are in early (Phase I or Phase II) clinical trial testing. A small proportion is being assessed in a Phase III setting and is being compared with the current best standard therapy.

New drugs that are in the advanced stages of clinical trial testing in pancreatic cancer include, but are not limited to, Pemetrexed, DX–8951f, MGI–114, Irinotecan, anti-*ras* agents (vaccines, oral and intravenous drugs), antiepidermal growth factor agents (e.g., Cetuximab and OSI–774), and antiangiogenic agents. This list is constantly changing, and for up-to-date information you should check with your treating oncologist or a reference academic medical center. For most of these drugs, it will be several years before definite answers are available with regard to value and/or superiority of these agents over standard therapy (which is currently single-agent gemcitabine for advanced pancreatic cancer).

Targeted therapies are a new class of drugs and vaccines that target a specific aspect of the cell cycle. Their benefit is that they may be more selective for certain characteristics of the cancer over normal cellular parts and, therefore, may result in fewer side effects. Multiple targeted-type therapies are being assessed in pancreatic cancer (e.g., OSI–774 and anti-*ras* agents; mentioned in the previous paragraph). For now, as a class, they remain an experimental treatment and have yet to prove reproducible activity in this disease. However, much of the hope for the future of pancreatic cancer is built on these types of agents.

If you are undergoing treatment at a medical institution that is offering one or more clinical trials, consider participating. Potentially very effective drugs are in the pipeline, and you might directly benefit from participation. Also, by doing so, you are contributing to the advancement of treatment options for pancreatic cancer patients.

PART FOUR

Managing Your Treatment

I don't feel that my doctor is explaining everything to me. How can I get answers to my questions?

How can I get a second opinion about my treatment?

More...

53. I don't feel that my doctor is explaining everything to me. How can I get answers to my questions?

You should feel comfortable and be able to communicate well with your doctor, and you should be able to trust his or her medical judgment. Doctors generally try to tell you everything that you need to know about your disease and treatment, but you may still have unanswered questions. Thus, you must first decide what you want to know.

You should feel comfortable and be able to communicate well with your doctor.

Everyone approaches a cancer diagnosis differently. Some people want to know every detail about their disease, treatment, and prognosis and will want to be involved in every decision that is made. Others prefer to know only the basics and to have their family or doctor make the decisions. Of course, many people fall in between. You will also likely want different information at various times, and your concerns will be different when you are first diagnosed than during or after your treatment. You may not even want to know some things at all. There is no right way to approach this; however, you need to decide how much you want to know and then discuss this with your family and doctor.

Decide what you want to learn before each doctor visit. Talk with family or friends to help focus your thoughts and concerns. Once you have clarified these, write down your specific questions. Be sure to include all of your concerns, as there are no silly questions. Tell your doctor at the beginning of the visit that you would like to ask some questions. The doctor will then likely plan extra time to speak with you. Here are some questions that you may want to ask:

There are no silly questions.

- Is the cancer localized, or has it spread to other sites?
- What other diagnostic tests do I need to have done?
- Can this cancer be surgically removed?
- What choices in treatment do I have?
- What treatment do you recommend and why?
- What is the goal of this treatment?
- What are the risks of this treatment?
- How will you know whether the treatment is working?
- What are the alternatives to this treatment?
- How will I feel during and after this treatment?
- What side effects will I have from this treatment?
- What do I need to do to care for myself during this treatment?
- Will I be able to work and continue my usual activities during treatment?
- For what reasons should I call your office?

In answering your questions, the doctor may have a lot of information and may use unfamiliar terms. You may feel uneasy or afraid as you listen and find it difficult to understand everything that is being said; if this happens, ask the doctor to explain further.

It is helpful to take notes while the doctor is speaking. You may even want to tape record the discussion or bring a family member or friend to listen to what is being said. Your companion can even take notes while the doctor is speaking and can review the answers with you at home. If something is still unclear when you get home, call the office. The nurse who works with your doctor may also be able to provide answers. You deserve to have responses to your questions; thus, it's okay to be persistent.

Although you may be more comfortable not knowing all of the details, family members may have many questions. It is a good idea to have one person be the family spokesperson, to possibly come to office visits and contact the doctor as needed to ask questions. The family spokesperson can use the same suggestions described previously here to ask and clarify everyone's questions.

54. I have heard that pancreatic cancer is one of the most dangerous. If my cancer cannot be cured, why should I get any treatment at all?

John's Comment:

Remember that any figure for 5-year mortality only considers patients who were diagnosed more than 5 years ago, and there have been significant advances in all areas of pancreatic cancer treatment within the past 5 to 10 years. As an excellent example, the drug gemcitabine (Gemzar) has only been employed as a chemotherapy agent for pancreatic cancer since 1996, and even today, not every oncologist and medical institution uses it. Although this disease remains one of the most serious of all cancers, every year the prospects for survival improve. A patient diagnosed today has a much better chance of full recovery than if diagnosed yesterday, and patients' chances could improve even more if any drugs that are now in clinical trials are shown to be effective.

Pancreatic cancer is one of the most difficult cancers to treat and can be cured only if it is diagnosed at a very early stage. Unfortunately, often no symptoms appear when the cancer first develops, and thus, by the time it is diagnosed it has often grown or spread and cannot be removed by surgery; nevertheless, it is important to remain hopeful.

One of the most difficult things about having cancer is living with uncertainty about the future. Some people want their doctor to predict what will happen to them and to give them statistics about their "chances." You should remember that these statistics represent averages that are seen in large numbers of people. Doctors cannot foresee what will happen to any one person. A statistic that is commonly reported is the percentage of people who are alive 5 years after being diagnosed. Of course, many people live much longer than 5 years. In pancreatic cancer, if the cancer has been completely removed, 12% to 20% of people will be alive at 5 years; however, when looking at all of the people diagnosed with pancreatic cancer, regardless of how much the cancer had spread when it was first diagnosed, only 2% to 4% will be alive 5 years later. You should remember that everyone is different and will thus respond differently to treatment. No one can predict precisely what will happen to you.

Even for those who cannot be cured, there are a number of benefits in obtaining treatment for pancreatic cancer. The disease can usually be controlled with treatment for a period of time, anywhere from months to years. Equally important to consider is that treatment can be very effective in improving the quality of your life. It can lessen or prevent symptoms of the disease, including pain, weight loss, and fatigue. In addition, it can prevent or put off complications that could develop if the cancer was allowed to grow without any attempt to control it. Many people with pancreatic cancer live full and satisfying lives.

One of the most difficult things about having cancer is living with uncertainty about the future.

Even for those who cannot be cured, there are a number of benefits in obtaining treatment.

Managing Your Treatment

55. How can I get a second opinion about my treatment?

The doctor who gave your initial diagnosis will probably recommend that you see an oncologist for treatment. After hearing an oncologist's recommendations, you may be interested in getting a second opinion. You need to determine what type of oncologist you want to see: a surgical oncologist (performs surgery), a medical oncologist (prescribes chemotherapy), or a radiation oncologist (prescribes radiation therapy). Before scheduling an appointment, you should check with your insurance company or Health Maintenance Organization to find out whether they provide reimbursement for second opinions.

The name(s) of an oncologist can be obtained in several ways: ask your doctor, contact your state medical society, contact a local academic hospital (one that is affiliated with a medical school), or contact the Cancer Information Service of the National Cancer Institute. Request to see someone who is board certified in his or her specialty and, if possible, someone who specializes in treating pancreatic or gastrointestinal cancers.

To ensure that you are able to get the most out of a second opinion visit, you need to bring all of your related medical information. Some doctors may even ask you to send this before your appointment. The things that you should have available include the following: (1) a pathology report that describes the type of cancer; (2) slides with samples of tissue from the tumor, obtained when you had your biopsy or surgery (you can get these from the department of pathology at the hospital where the procedure was done); (3) if you had surgery, the report describing the surgery performed; (4) any scans or MRIs that were performed (the actual images as well as copies of the reports); (5) a description of any treatments that you have had thus far; (6) a list of all of the medications that you are currently taking, including over-the-counter medications, nutritional supplements, herbs, and vitamins; and (7) any other relevant medical reports that you have available.

The doctor that you see for a second opinion will review all of your medical information. You shouldn't be surprised that the doctor wants to take a complete history and perform a physical exam, even though you have gone through all of this before. The doctor will want to be sure that he or she has all of the important information and that nothing has been missed, and he or she may even recommend that additional diagnostic tests be done. After analyzing all of this information, the doctor should explain what treatment options are available and recommend what will be best for you.

John's Comment:

Before you select a particular doctor or institution for your treatment, you must ask them this: "What is your personal experience treating patients with pancreatic cancer? How many patients? With what results?" Because pancreatic cancer isn't all that prevalent, many—if not most—oncologists and surgeons have little or no experience in treating the disease. This is particularly critical when selecting a surgeon and a hospital should you qualify for surgery. You want to have the best, most experienced professionals as your team, employing the very latest techniques and drugs for radiotherapy and chemotherapy and surgical procedures. The most highly regarded cancer centers may offer you the very best chance of success, and if it's at all feasible, you should get to one of them quickly!

56. What are complementary and alternative treatments?

Complementary and alternative medicine, also referred to as **integrative medicine**, refers to a variety of approaches that improve health and treat disease that the traditional medical community does not recognize as standard. When used in addition to conventional methods of treatment, they are referred to as complementary; when used instead of conventional methods of treatment, they are referred to as alternative.

Complementary and alternative therapies may be categorized in many different ways. The National Center for Complementary and Alternative Medicine divides them into five domains:

- Alternative medical systems of theory and practice. Many of these are used by different cultures in various parts of the world (e.g., Asian, Indian, and Native American Indian practices). Acupuncture originated as a part of traditional Chinese medicine. Other examples of alternative medical systems are homeopathic and naturopathic medicines.
- Mind–body interventions. These techniques help the mind to enhance various body functions and to reduce symptoms. Examples include relaxation, meditation, guided imagery, hypnosis, prayer, and support groups.
- Biologic-based therapies. These include dietary (e.g., the Gonzales diet and the macrobiotic diet), herbal (e.g., saw palmetto), biologic (e.g., shark cartilage), and orthomolecular (e.g., vitamins) treatments.

Integrative medicine

the use of complementary or alternative therapies, a variety of approaches to improve health and treat disease that are not recognized as standard by the traditional medical community.

- Manipulative and body-based methods. These techniques involve manipulation or movement of the body, such as those used by chiropractors and massage therapists.
- Energy therapies. These techniques manipulate energy fields within or outside of the body, such as therapeutic touch, Reiki, or magnets.

The use of complementary and alternative therapies is rapidly increasing, partially because of our increasing understanding of them. There is a constantly growing body of scientific knowledge about specific complementary and alternative therapies, how they work, and what effects they have on the body. The U.S. government, to spread reliable information about complementary and alternative therapies and to scientifically study their safety and effectiveness, recently founded the National Center for Complementary and Alternative Medicine as part of the National Institutes of Health.

The increased use of complementary and alternative therapies, however, also reflects the fact that many people with cancer are fearful and thus willing to try anything and everything that they feel may be helpful. Complementary and alternative therapies are not regulated in the same way that medications and medical devices are. Many treatments and products can be purchased for which there is no evidence of usefulness. In fact, some of these may even harm you. If you are considering one of these therapies, it is important to get a lot of accurate information. You should discuss your thoughts with your doctor and inform him or her of your plans. Many of these therapies can be used safely with the traditional treatments that you are receiving; however, some can interfere with your treatment, be

It is important to get a lot of accurate information.

harmful to you, or cause serious side effects when combined with your treatment.

57. How can I find out about complementary and alternative therapies?

Several reliable sources provide information about complementary and alternative therapies. Because of the rapidly changing state of knowledge about this area of medicine, the Internet provides the most up-to-date information. Resources with general information on complementary and alternative therapies include:

- Cancer Information Service of the National Cancer Institute (*cis.nci.nih.gov/fact/9_14.htm*)
- National Center for Complementary and Alternative Medicine of the National Institutes of Health (*nccam.nih.gov/fcp/factsheets/index.html*)
- The Richard and Hinda Rosenthal Center for Complementary and Alternative Medicine at Columbia University (*cpmcnet.columbia.edu/dept/rosenthal/CAM_Resources.html*)
- MD Anderson Complementary/Integrative Medicine Education Resources (*mdanderson.org/departments/ CIMER/*)
- Oncolink, from the University of Pennsylvania (*oncolink.upenn.edu/templates/treatment/index.cfm*).

Resources with information specifically about dietary supplements, including vitamins, minerals, and botanicals, include:

- Office of Dietary Supplements of the National Institutes of Health (*dietary-supplements.info.nih.gov/databases/ibids.html*)

- Center for Food Safety and Applied Nutrition of the U.S. Food and Drug Administration (*www. cfsan.fda.gov/~dms/ds-oview.html*)
- American Botanical Council (*www.herbalgram.org*)
- Supplement Watch (*supplementwatch.com*)
- Quackwatch (*Quackwatch.com*).

For scientific bibliographic citations related to particular therapies, see the following:

- National Library of Medicine (*www.nlm.nih.gov/ nccam/camonpubmed.html*).

58. How do I decide whether I should use one of the complementary or alternative therapies that my family or friends are recommending?

Before beginning treatment, obtain as much information as you can about the complementary or alternative therapy (Question 57). Some specific questions to consider are as follows:

- Do the promises sound too good to be true (e.g., promises of cure that are inconsistent with the information that you are receiving from your doctor or from other sources of information)?
- What is the evidence supporting the claims of effectiveness? Were scientific, controlled clinical trials conducted, or is the evidence only anecdotal, based on the author's personal experience or claims of satisfied customers?
- What are the risks of using this treatment? What is the evidence of the treatment's safety? How were the safety data collected?

- If a particular person is providing the therapy, what are his or her qualifications, certifications, or licenses? Some practitioners are now licensed by state medical boards or accredited by professional organizations.
- Is the source of information about the therapy also the seller of the therapy? If that is the case, they may have a financial interest in convincing you to purchase the product.

Two Internet sites provide tips to help make decisions about using a complementary or alternative therapy:

- National Center for Complementary and Alternative Medicine of the National Institutes of Health (*nccam.nih.gov/fcp/faq/considercam.htm*)
- Center for Food Safety and Applied Nutrition of the U.S. Food and Drug Administration (*www.cfsan.fda.gov/~dms/ds-savvy.html*).

Before making a final decision about the use of any complementary or alternative therapy, discuss your thoughts with your doctor and inform him or her of your intentions. Many of these therapies can be used safely with the traditional treatments that you are receiving. However, some can interfere with your treatment, cause serious side effects when combined with your treatment, or be harmful to you.

59. So much information is available on the Internet. How do I evaluate this information to be sure that it is complete, accurate, and up-to-date?

You can get instant access via the Internet to an enormous amount of information without ever leaving your home. You can use the Internet to obtain information about pancreatic cancer and its treatment; however, you should remember that because there is no control or regulation of the information that is posted on the Internet, much of it may not be accurate.

When viewing a particular site, you should look for specific elements to determine whether the site is reliable and likely to have complete, accurate, and up-to-date information, including the following:

- Owner or sponsor of the site. The owner or sponsor of the site (a government agency, a nonprofit organization, a medical center or hospital, a pharmaceutical company, or an individual) pays for it to be maintained and thus can influence what content is presented. You should consider whether the sponsor could benefit by presenting a biased point of view.
- Purpose of the site. The purpose of the site is usually found by clicking "About This Site." It should be clearly stated and will help to determine whether there is a particular point of view.
- Editorial board. Many sites have an editorial board that reviews all of the information posted on the web site. Review the list of people on the editorial board and check their credentials and affiliations to be sure that they are medically qualified to make these decisions.
- Source of information. The author of the information should be identified. Review the credentials and affiliations of the author to be sure that he or she is truly an expert in the field. Other sources for the information should be acknowledged.
- Evidence. References to scientific research findings and published articles that back up the information should be included.

- Date the information was updated. The site should include a statement indicating the date that the information was last reviewed and updated. Medical information must be current to be useful.
- Privacy. The site may ask you for personal information. It should clearly state how the information will be used and how your privacy will be protected.

Before acting on any information that you get from the Internet, discuss your findings and considerations with your doctor.

John's Comment:

The Internet is a very helpful tool. When I was diagnosed, I knew next to nothing about the functions of the pancreas, let alone what pancreatic cancer was all about. I found it very efficient to obtain basic information from a variety of public service web sites and to research which medical institutions had a focus on and significant experience with this disease.

PART FIVE

Changes Cancer Brings

I feel so overwhelmed by all of the information that I am getting. How do I make decisions about my treatment?

My doctor told me that I should take pancreatic enzymes. What are these, and why do I need to take them?

More ...

60. I feel so overwhelmed by all of the information that I am getting. How do I make decisions about my treatment?

Joy's Comment:

When I was first diagnosed and upon learning that the surgery was called "Whipple," a friend looked up information on it for me. Everything was so negative (and out of date) on the Whipple procedure—and there was so little good news on pancreatic cancer—that I stopped doing research. I had the Whipple in January 2000 and it wasn't until January 2001 (when my Ca19-9 started rising) that I started researching again. I didn't know about the Johns Hopkins pancreatic cancer web site—with its remarkable online chat room—or PanCAN. It's difficult to say in retrospect whether I would have wanted to know more at the early stage or not as there is hardly any good news, but more than 2.5 years later, I'm still here and doing good. I've since become acquainted via PanCAN and e-mail with many "long-term" survivors—most who have had the Whipple, but some who haven't had surgery. My outlook is that there's no reason I shouldn't be one of the good statistics!

After being diagnosed with cancer, one of the most stressful periods is when you have to make decisions about your treatment. A number of things can help you sort out the options and select the one that is best for you.

First, you need to be sure that you have all of the relevant information. Are you clear about your clinical situation and the choices that are being presented to you? (Question 53 gives you a list of questions to ask your doctor to help you understand your situation.) Second, you should see all of the treating specialists to hear their recommendations directly. An internist or surgeon can provide you with direction, but he or she will not be able to give you detailed information about chemotherapy or radiation therapy. If these treatments are being recommended, schedule appointments with a medical oncologist (who prescribes chemotherapy) and a radiation oncologist (who prescribes radiation therapy). Each doctor should clarify the goals of treatment. Ask also about the potential side effects or risks of treatment (see Question 53 for additional questions that you may want to ask). This will help you analyze the choices.

Once you are clear on the options that the doctors are giving you, consider whether it is worthwhile to get a second opinion, perhaps with a specialist at an academic center or comprehensive cancer center (Question 55). Doctors who specialize in treating pancreatic cancer or other gastrointestinal cancers have more experience with this disease and may have a different viewpoint about treatment. In addition, they may be able to offer treatment in a clinical trial for people with pancreatic cancer.

It will be helpful to have a family member or friend go with you to these appointments, as they can also hear the information and even take notes while the doctors are speaking. When you get home, this person can review all of the information to be sure that you understand it correctly.

It will be helpful to have a family member or friend go with you to these appointments.

In making your final treatment decision, several other factors need to be considered. Financial issues are important. What are the costs of the various treatment options, including treatment on a clinical trial? Does your health insurance cover treatment by any doctor or only by the doctors that are affiliated with your health insurance plan? Will treatment on a clinical trial be covered? What percentage of the costs are reimbursed to you, and what are the out-of-pocket expenses? Logistical issues are also important. Where would you have to go for treatment? Will it be easy to get back and forth, or will you have to travel long distances or even move to a different city for a period of time? Finally, it is important to consider your emotional reactions toward the different doctors that you have met. Did you feel that you could trust the doctor? Did you feel that you were given adequate time to have all of your questions answered? Did the staff in the office treat you respectfully and courteously? It is important to feel comfortable with the doctor that you choose because he or she will be your partner in the journey that lies ahead.

In the end, the decision is yours. Consider everything about your current life situation: your age; your general state of health; your responsibilities regarding family and work; the emotional, physical, and financial costs of treatment; and all that you may possibly gain from treatment. The most difficult part of this process is that there is no "right" decision waiting to be found, only the one that feels right to you.

Joy's Comment:

The Johns Hopkins chat room on their web site is a good place to ask for recommendations. These are people who have had personal experience with numerous doctors. Also, PanCAN has the names of doctors who specialize in pancreatic cancer (see the Appendix).

61. After surgery, I frequently get diarrhea and cramps. My doctor told me that I should take pancreatic enzymes. What are these, and why do I need to take them?

One function of the pancreas is to secrete digestive enzymes that break down the food that you eat into basic nutrients that the body can absorb. Normally, the pancreas adjusts the amount of enzymes secreted based on what you eat. When you have cancer of the pancreas, or after a surgery in which part or all of your pancreas is removed, you may no longer secrete an adequate amount of pancreatic enzymes (**pancreatic insufficiency**). As a result, the food that you eat does not get fully digested. As it passes through the intestine, the food cannot get absorbed, and it pulls water into the intestine, causing cramping and diarrhea. You may also notice frequent bowel movements that look oily or greasy and float in the toilet. If this persists for a long time, you may lose weight because of the lack of nutrients.

Pancreatic insufficiency
inability of the pancreas to secrete an adequate amount of enzymes needed to digest food.

Taking pancreatic enzymes by mouth each time that you eat can prevent these problems. Pancreatic enzymes are available in capsule or tablet form. Your doctor can prescribe these for you. Generally, people take one to two capsules as they start eating and may take one to two more about 10 to 15 minutes into the meal, trying to mimic what happens naturally in the body. If your starting dose does not control the cramping or diarrhea, tell your doctor or nurse. They will adjust the dose until your symptoms are controlled. You may need less when just eating a snack or more when eating a meal high in fat (e.g., fried foods, cheeses, fatty meats, gravies, or cream sauces). The enzymes come in varying strengths, and thus, if you find that you need to take many during each meal, ask your doctor for a more concentrated dose.

John's Comment:

I take pancreatic enzymes with every meal—or at least I'm supposed to! Sometimes I forget to take them, but I do not notice any difference in how I feel, nor do I experience any symptoms when I forget. That must mean that the 60% of my pancreas that remains is getting the job done. And I eat everything in sight! I also take Prevacid and Celebrex daily.

Joy's Comment:

I always have taken enzymes, but I didn't know there were different kinds. Be sure if you continue to have frequent "fatty" bowel movements to ask your doctor about different enzymes.

62. After surgery, my doctor told me that I might develop diabetes. Why does this happen and what should I do to check for and treat this?

One function of the pancreas is to secrete insulin into the blood stream. Insulin enables glucose (a form of sugar) to be transported into your cells, giving you energy throughout the day. Normally, the pancreas adjusts the amount of insulin secreted based on what you eat and on your activity level. When you have cancer of the pancreas, or after pancreatic surgery in which part or all of your pancreas is removed, you may no longer secrete the correct amount of insulin, or your body may become partially resistant to insulin. The glucose is not able to enter your cells effectively, and the level of glucose in your blood rises, which is called hyperglycemia. Diabetes is persistent hyperglycemia. Signs or symptoms of diabetes include frequent urination, thirst, fatigue, blurred vision, and weight loss.

Your doctor will periodically check your blood chemistries, including the glucose level. If you develop persistent hyperglycemia, you may be referred to an endocrinologist, a doctor who specializes in hormonal diseases, including diabetes. Additional blood tests may be ordered, and the best treatment for you will be determined. This may involve a change in diet and an increase in exercise. You may also have to take either oral medication or insulin, which is injected under your skin. It is important to treat diabetes to prevent long-term complications, which can result in heart and blood vessel disease, strokes, and visual, kidney, and neurologic problems.

63. Is it true that radiation therapy causes a skin reaction? How should I care for my skin during radiation therapy?

Radiation therapy is administered as a beam of energy directed from a treatment machine at precise angles toward a defined target in your body. It destroys tumor cells in its path by preventing them from dividing. Normal cells that divide rapidly are also very sensitive to the effects of radiation therapy. As a result, changes may be seen in your skin where the beam enters and exits your body. When receiving radiation therapy for pancreatic cancer, the skin changes occur most commonly on the abdomen and middle of the back. You may notice redness, tanning, dryness, flaking, and/or itching. These are all normal effects of radiation that generally begin about 2 weeks after you start treatment and that last for about 1 month after treatment is completed. After that, you may have an area of darkened skin on your abdomen or back.

Radiation therapy to the abdomen does not cause a loss of hair on the head, but if you have hair on your abdomen or back, you may notice that the hair falls out in this area. It will grow back several months after your treatment is completed.

Taking special care of your skin from the first day of treatment will ensure that you do not become uncomfortable from the changes that occur. Bathe daily using warm water and a mild, nonperfumed soap. Do not scrub the skin with a cloth or brush, rinse the soap entirely, and gently pat the skin dry. Your doctor or nurse may recommend using a moisturizer (e.g., aloe vera gel or Aquaphor) either from the beginning of treatment or if you develop dryness or itching. Most commonly, it's recommended that you use these twice a day: after your daily treatment and at bedtime. Check before using any other lotions, creams, or ointments in the area being treated, as some products can make the skin reaction more severe.

You should also avoid irritating the skin in the treated area, the abdomen, and middle back. Specific suggestions for this part of the body include avoiding the following: tight clothing, use of tape, scratching the skin (tell your doctor or nurse if the moisturizers are not effective in relieving the itching so that something else can be prescribed), direct sunlight, and the use of ice packs or heating pads.

64. Will chemotherapy cause hair loss? Can I prevent this? What can I do to feel good about my appearance?

Chemotherapy destroys tumor cells by preventing them from dividing. Normal cells that divide rapidly are very sensitive to the effects of chemotherapy. The cells at the base of the hair may become unable to divide to make new cells, weakening the hair shaft and resulting in loss of hair. Some people experience only a thinning of their hair, but some people lose all of the hair on their head. Certain chemotherapy drugs are much more likely than others to cause hair loss. Your doctor or nurse can tell you whether you are likely to lose your hair based on the type of chemotherapy drug that you are receiving. If you are receiving chemotherapy drugs that are likely to cause hair loss, it is also possible that you will lose hair in other parts of your body, including your eyebrows, eyelashes, underarm, and pubic hair. Hair loss usually begins about 3 weeks after chemotherapy begins. Sometimes people notice a gradual thinning and loss of hair, but with some chemotherapy agents, the hair can come out in clumps over a period of only a few days.

If you are receiving chemotherapy that causes only a thinning of hair, these suggestions may reduce the amount of hair that you lose: use mild shampoos (e.g., baby shampoo), use a soft-bristled hairbrush, avoid permanents and hair dyes, and avoid heated rollers and high-heat hair dryers.

If you are receiving chemotherapy that has a high likelihood of causing complete hair loss, there is no way of preventing this. We no longer use ice caps to prevent the chemotherapy from flowing to the scalp, as we want to be sure the chemotherapy travels all over your body without missing any area where there could be cancer cells.

If your doctor or nurse tells you that there is a high likelihood that you will lose your hair from treatment, you may find it helpful to purchase a wig or hairpiece before you lose your hair. Some people like to match their own hairstyle to maintain their usual appearance, but others like to try a new look. Wigs can be made from human hair or synthetic fibers and vary considerably in price. Stores in your area might specialize in working with people who lose their hair from cancer treatment, or you can also purchase a wig or hairpiece through the American Cancer Society. Your local American Cancer Society or hospital social work department may also have wigs and hairpieces that can be loaned. Your insurance company may reimburse the cost of a wig or hairpiece. Check your policy, and if this is covered, ask your doctor to give you a prescription for a "hair prosthesis needed for cancer treatment."

Some people prefer to wear a turban, scarf, or cap to cover their head, and some people prefer to leave their head uncovered. You should do whatever makes you feel the most comfortable (but be careful to protect your scalp from sunburn if you go without a head covering). It is important to not let your changed appearance modify your interactions with family, friends, and coworkers. Despite the loss of hair, you can do many things to feel good about your appearance (e.g., taking care in the clothes you wear, using makeup, and wearing beautiful scarves). In addition, the American

Cancer Society and the Cosmetic, Toiletry, and Fragrance Association sponsor a free program—"Look Good, Feel Better"—that is dedicated to helping women who have cancer feel better about their appearance. They teach beauty techniques that help restore appearance and enhance self-image. To find out whether it is available in your area, go to their Internet site (*www.lookgoodfeelbetter.org*) or call your local American Cancer Society office.

65. I have heard that chemotherapy may cause sores in my mouth. How should I care for my mouth during chemotherapy?

Chemotherapy destroys tumor cells by preventing them from dividing. Normal cells that divide rapidly are also sensitive to the effects of chemotherapy. With certain chemotherapy drugs, the mucous membranes that line the inside of your mouth and throat may be affected and may become reddened and feel tender, sore, or painful. You may even develop sores or ulcers in the mouth or throat or have difficulty swallowing. This is called **stomatitis**, and some chemotherapy drugs, such as 5-FU, are much more likely than others to cause stomatitis. If you develop severe stomatitis, your doctor may reduce the dose of chemotherapy for your next treatment. Radiation therapy to the abdomen does not cause stomatitis.

Many effective ways of managing sores in the mouth are available. First, it is important to keep your mouth clean and moist to prevent infection. Brush your teeth with a soft-bristled toothbrush after each meal and rinse regularly with a saltwater solution. You can add

Stomatitis
inflammation of the mucous membranes of the mouth from chemotherapy; may be associated with sores, ulcers, and mouth pain.

Keep your mouth clean and moist to prevent infection.

table salt or baking soda to a glass of warm water and then swish and spit. Do not use a commercial mouthwash because most contain alcohol, which can irritate your mouth. If your mouth or throat becomes sore or painful, let your doctor or nurse know so that a medication can be prescribed. You can swish topical anesthetic medications in your mouth to numb the membranes, but if your mouth is very painful, a narcotic medication may be more helpful. If your lips become irritated, A&D ointment may be soothing.

Changes in what you eat and drink may also help to manage stomatitis. Some specific suggestions include the following:

- Eat soft or pureed foods that are easy to chew and swallow.
- If you are having difficulty swallowing solid foods, drink liquid nutritional supplements that are available in your local drugstore. Your doctor or nurse can recommend specific supplements for you.
- Avoid hot foods or liquids.
- Avoid foods and liquids that can irritate the membranes (e.g., alcohol, citrus, tomatoes, spices, and rough coarse foods).
- Avoid smoking.

If you are having difficulty swallowing your medications, ask your doctor to prescribe a liquid version if it is available. If a liquid version is not available, many medications can be crushed and mixed with a small amount of juice or applesauce to make them easier to swallow. Check with your pharmacist before crushing, however, as this may affect the way the medication works.

66. What can I do to prevent or relieve nausea and vomiting related to my chemotherapy or radiation therapy?

Nausea and vomiting have long been considered to be unavoidable side effects of cancer treatment; however, with the development in recent years of new antinausea medications (antiemetics), this is no longer the case. Both radiation therapy to the abdominal area and chemotherapy may cause nausea or vomiting. This can result from irritation of the stomach or from chemical stimulation of areas in the brain that trigger nausea and vomiting. Vomiting is when you throw up stomach contents through your mouth. Retching, gagging, or dry heaves feel similar to vomiting, but no stomach contents come up.

Whether you develop nausea or vomiting depends on many things, including what chemotherapy drugs you are getting. The most commonly used chemotherapy drugs (gemcitabine and 5-FU) for treating cancer of the pancreas cause nausea or vomiting in 10% to 30% of people if they receive no antinausea medication. With radiation therapy to the abdominal area, approximately 50% of people experience nausea or vomiting if they receive no antinausea medication. With medication, the likelihood that you will experience nausea or vomiting with either treatment is much lower.

People vary widely in their reactions to the same treatment: Some have very distressing symptoms, others mild symptoms, and yet others no nausea or vomiting at all. For people who do experience nausea or vomiting, the timing of the symptoms will also vary. Some patients develop symptoms within minutes or hours after treatment, and some develop symptoms days later. For some patients the symptoms may last several hours, and for others they may last for many days. Certain patients have the most severe symptoms before leaving home in the morning or while on their way to treatment; this is called "anticipatory" nausea or vomiting.

Nausea and vomiting can be prevented or well controlled in most people.

Many effective ways of managing nausea and vomiting are available, but the most important is the use of medication. Several new antinausea medications have been developed in recent years, and as we have learned new ways of using and combining these medications, nausea and vomiting can be prevented or well controlled in most people. These medications are most commonly given orally, intravenously, or by a suppository inserted into the rectum. Depending on the specific treatment that you are getting and on the timing and severity of your symptoms, your doctor will prescribe a specific antinausea medication for you. You may be instructed to take the medication at home before coming for treatment. The nurse may give you medication immediately before your chemotherapy, or you may be instructed to take the medication on a schedule at home after your treatment. Different antinausea medications work in different ways; thus, if one medication is not effective, call your doctor or nurse and ask for another medication because nausea and vomiting can be effectively treated.

Other ways besides medication are also available for managing nausea or vomiting. Techniques that use your body and mind can be very helpful, particularly with anticipatory nausea or vomiting (e.g., guided imagery, self-hypnosis, and progressive muscle relaxation). Ask your doctor or nurse for a referral to someone trained in these techniques if you are interested in learning one of them. Also, some people find it helpful to minimize the use of things in the home that have particularly strong odors (e.g., perfumes or certain cleaning products).

Changes in what you eat and drink may also help to manage nausea and vomiting. Some specific suggestions include the following:

- Eat a light meal before each treatment.
- Eat small amounts of food and liquids at a time.
- Eat bland foods and liquids.
- Eat dry crackers when feeling nauseated.
- Limit the amount of liquids that you take with your meals.
- Maintain adequate liquids between meals, taking mostly clear liquids such as water, apple juice, herbal tea, or bullion (some people find that carbonated sodas are helpful; others do better to drink soda without the fizz).
- Eat cool foods or foods at room temperature.
- Avoid foods with strong odors.
- Avoid high-fat, greasy, and fried foods.
- Avoid spicy foods, alcohol, and caffeine.

A nutritionist can help you to select appropriate foods. Ask your doctor or nurse for a referral. Taking in enough fluids and nutrients is important for your health. If you are unable to keep any food or liquids down for 12 hours or if you are taking in only small amounts of food or liquids for 24 hours, call your doctor or nurse.

67. What can I do for diarrhea related to radiation therapy or chemotherapy?

Chemotherapy and radiation therapy destroy tumor cells by preventing them from dividing. Normal cells that divide rapidly are also very sensitive to the effects of these treatments. The small intestine lies within the radiation therapy treatment field, and thus, the mucous membranes that line the small intestine become thinner and lose their ability to function as effectively as normal. As a result, the intestines do not absorb fluid and nutrients adequately and do not digest lactose (the sugar in milk) well. In addition, the muscle layer of the intestine becomes overactive, moving the intestinal contents through the bowel more quickly than usual. All of this may result in abdominal cramping and diarrhea. Some chemotherapy drugs (e.g., 5-FU) are much more likely than others to cause diarrhea.

Many effective ways of managing cramping and diarrhea are available. Antidiarrheal medications such as Imodium AD (available over the counter) or Lomotil (requires a prescription) are very effective. Follow your doctor's or nurse's instructions on how to take these medications.

Changes in what you eat and drink will also help to manage diarrhea. Some specific suggestions include the following:

• Eat small amounts of food and liquids at a time.
• Eat bland foods and liquids.
• Increase the amount of fluid you drink when having diarrhea.

- Drink a variety of liquids that you can see through (e.g., apple juice, cranberry juice, herbal teas, and Jell-O).
- Sports drinks with electrolytes are particularly good, as well as fat-free broth or bullion.
- Avoid liquids with alcohol and caffeine.
- Avoid high-fiber foods.
- Avoid whole-grain breads and cereals. Instead, try to eat white bread, pasta, noodles, cold cereals of corn or rice, saltines, and white rice.
- Avoid raw fruits and vegetables, cooked vegetables that cause gas, and beans. Instead, you should have bananas, applesauce, canned cooked fruits with skin removed, white potatoes without the skin, cooked squash or carrots, and tomato paste or puree (without chunks of tomato). Bananas and white potatoes are good sources of potassium, which is important to replace if you have diarrhea.
- Avoid foods high in lactose (e.g., milk, ice cream, and soft cheeses). Drink lactose-free milk and eat hard cheeses, yogurt, and sorbet.
- Avoid fatty, greasy, and fried foods, including cream sauces and gravies, and limit the amount of butter and oil that you use.

A nutritionist can help you to select appropriate foods. Ask your doctor or nurse for a referral. Taking in enough fluid and nutrients is important for good health. You can become severely dehydrated if you have severe diarrhea and are not able to replace the fluid that you lose. If your diarrhea does not respond within 12 hours to the medications that you are taking and to changes in your diet, call your doctor or nurse.

68. I was told that chemotherapy may cause a drop in my blood counts. What does this mean?

Bone marrow

substance in the center of many bones where blood cells are produced.

Blood cells are produced in the **bone marrow** and are then released into the blood stream where they protect the body in a variety of ways. White cells fight infection. Platelets stop bleeding by clumping together to plug damaged blood vessels. Red cells carry oxygen from the lungs to all of the tissues of the body, where the cells use it to create energy. Testing a blood sample for the number of cells in the blood can be done; this is called a complete blood count. The number of red cells is also reflected in measurements called hematocrit (the percentage of red cells in the blood) and hemoglobin (the amount of the molecule in the red cells that carries the oxygen). The normal ranges for a complete blood count vary from lab to lab, but in general, normal values are as follows: white blood cells, 4000 to 10,000 cells/mm^3; platelets, 150,000 to 500,000 cells/mm^3; hemoglobin, 12 to 18 g/dL; and hematocrit, 36% to 54%.

Blood cells only live for a short time after they are released into the bloodstream: 24 hours for some types of white cells, about 10 days for platelets, and about 3 months for red cells. The body depends on the rapidly dividing cells in the bone marrow to continuously replace these cells as they die.

Chemotherapy destroys tumor cells by preventing them from dividing. Normal cells that divide rapidly are very sensitive to the effects of chemotherapy. The cells in the bone marrow lose their ability to form new blood cells; thus, fewer cells are released into the blood stream. The blood counts drop after chemotherapy is given, generally 7 to 14 days after treatment. The white cells and platelets are particularly sensitive because they live for only a short period of time. The body can adjust to slight decreases in the number of blood cells without any problem; however, your doctor will order blood tests before you get each cycle of chemotherapy to be sure that your counts are not too low. If they are, your treatment may be stopped for a week to give the bone marrow a chance to make new blood cells.

69. What happens if my blood counts are too low? How should I take care of myself?

If the white cell count drops, you have an increased risk of developing an infection. Throughout your treatment, you can do certain things to prevent infection:

- Wash your hands frequently with soap and water, especially before eating and after going to the bathroom.
- Bathe daily with soap and water, and brush your teeth after each meal.
- Limit contact with people who have colds or flu.
- Avoid sharing food utensils, drinking glasses, or toothbrushes.
- Avoid handling feces or urine of pets, especially in cat litter or birdcage droppings.
- Check with your doctor or nurse before receiving any dental work or immunizations.

If your white cell counts drop very low, you may be advised to take precautions to prevent infection. In addition, your doctor may recommend a medication called filgrastim (Neupogen), which stimulates the bone marrow to make new white cells quickly. It is injected under your skin with a small thin needle once a day until your white blood cell count comes up. You or a family member can be taught how to give the injection at home.

Despite doing everything correctly, you may still develop an infection. If you have a biliary stent in place to open a blockage of the bile duct (see Question 21), you have a higher than normal risk of developing an infection. You will not feel that your counts are low, and thus, you should call your doctor or nurse if you have any symptoms of infection: fever of 100.5°F or 38°C; shaking chills; sore throat or cough; increased frequency or burning when you urinate; swelling, redness, or pain anywhere on your skin; and vomiting or diarrhea unrelated to your chemotherapy.

If the platelet count drops, you have an increased risk of bleeding. Throughout your treatment, avoid aspirin, products that contain aspirin, and nonsteroidal anti-inflammatory drugs such as ibuprofen, as these may all affect platelet function. If the platelet counts drop very low, you may be advised to take precautions to prevent bleeding, such as using only an electric razor and avoiding activities in which you could be injured.

Because you will not feel that your counts are low, you should call your doctor or nurse if you develop any signs of bleeding, including easy bruising, bleeding gums or nose bleeds, blood in the urine or stool, and black stools.

If the red cell count drops, you will feel fatigued (e.g., a lack of energy; feeling tired, weak, or weary; feeling irritable or depressed; or having difficulty concentrating). You may even feel lightheaded or short of breath

(Question 70 discusses how to conserve energy and manage fatigue).

If your red cell counts fall very low, your doctor may recommend a medication called epoetin (Procrit, Epogen), which stimulates the bone marrow to make more red cells. It is injected under the skin with a very small thin needle and can be given either three times or once a week. Some people give themselves the injection; others get it from their oncology nurse. You may also be instructed to take an oral iron supplement while getting these injections.

70. I feel tired much of the time. What can I do to increase my energy?

Fatigue is a common problem for people with cancer and causes you to feel tired, weak, or weary; lack energy; be unable to concentrate; or feel irritable or depressed. Many things can cause fatigue: the disease itself, the treatment that you are receiving, the side effects of certain medications (e.g., medications to treat pain or nausea), anemia (low red blood cell count), a decrease in the amount of food that you eat, a decrease in the amount of liquids that you drink, difficulty sleeping, emotional distress, and chronic pain. However, many people with cancer develop fatigue without any clear single cause.

Fatigue is a common problem for people with cancer.

Sleeping extra hours at night by going to bed earlier or staying in bed a bit later in the morning will improve your energy. Resting (napping for short periods or just laying down and relaxing) during the day is also important. Plan these rest periods when you know that you will be more likely to feel tired. For some people, even bathing, dressing, or eating may cause tiredness, and it is helpful to rest after these activities. However, at the same time, you should push yourself to be as active as possible. Lying in bed all day will generally make you weaker. In fact, evidence exists that exercising will actually increase your energy level as long as you don't push yourself to the point of exhaustion. If you are currently exercising on a regular basis, try to maintain this, but adjust the amount and frequency of your exercise routine based on how you feel. If you are not currently exercising, take a daily walk—starting with 5 to 15 minutes a day and adjusting the distance and speed based on how you feel. The key thing is finding a balance between rest and activity.

Exercising will actually increase your energy level.

Anemia causes fatigue. Epoetin (Procrit, Epogen), can treat anemia by stimulating your bone marrow to make more red blood cells (Question 69).

Anemia

low red blood cell counts.

If you have other specific problems that you think may be adding to your fatigue, speak with your doctor or nurse about these. Ask about taking a sleeping medication if you are not sleeping well, about how to better manage your pain if you are not comfortable, about how you can better cope with your emotional distress, and about how to increase your food and fluid intake if you feel you aren't taking in enough. Unfortunately, fatigue cannot always be effectively treated. It is often necessary to adjust your activity level to the changes in your energy level.

Save your energy for those things that are most important to you.

It is important to save your energy for those things that are most important to you. You need to think about all of the things that you do during the day: work, shopping, cooking, cleaning, household chores, errands, taking care of children or dependent relatives, being with family and friends, and recreational or leisure activities. Which of these activities are most important to you? Which give you the most pleasure? Which make you feel good about yourself? These are the things for which you will want to save your energy. You will probably notice that your energy level is greater at certain times of the day. Plan these activities for those times. For the other things that must get done, ask family and friends for help. People often want to help but don't know how. Tell them specifically what you need; they will probably be grateful for the direction (see Question 90 for suggestions on how family and friends can help). Finally, let go of the things that you don't need or want to do.

71. I have difficulty sleeping at night. What can I do to sleep better and feel more rested?

Difficulty falling asleep in the evening or difficulty staying asleep throughout the night are common problems for people with pancreatic cancer. Aside from the distress of lying awake in bed for many hours, not getting enough sleep may cause you to feel irritable and tired throughout the day and to have difficulty concentrating.

First try to determine the causes of your sleeplessness. Are you physically uncomfortable or in pain? Are you having other symptoms (e.g., nausea, vomiting, diarrhea, constipation, itching, mouth sores) that are making it difficult to sleep? To get a restful night's sleep, it is very important to take medication as prescribed to treat these problems. If you are taking medication and it is not effective, tell your doctor or nurse.

Are you feeling anxious and worried during the night? Are your thoughts racing and keeping you awake at night? Speaking with someone whom you trust and feel supported by about your thoughts and feelings may provide a significant amount of relief (see Question 81). For some people, medication for anxiety may be helpful.

Do you feel generally restless at night and unable to relax and sleep? A variety of techniques may be helpful:

- Establish a regular time to go to bed each night.
- Even if you do not sleep well at night, try not to sleep too much during the day. This will disrupt your body's normal cycle. If you are very tired, take only a short nap during the day (about 1 hour).
- Avoid being in bed at any time except when you are going to sleep. When resting during the day, lay in another room, on a couch or chair. Use your bed only for sleep at night.
- Avoid drinking caffeine or stimulants after dinner.
- Try a method of relaxation (see Question 57).

For some people, these techniques are still not helpful. If you continue to have difficulty sleeping, ask your doctor to prescribe a sleeping medication. Getting a restful sleep will help you to feel energized and capable during the day.

72. Will I have pain? What options are available to treat my pain?

Pain has long been considered to be an unavoidable consequence of having cancer, particularly cancer of the pancreas; however, with the development in recent years of new pain medications and with increasing understanding of how to use these more effectively, cancer pain can be adequately controlled in almost all people.

Without any medication, many people with pancreatic cancer will have pain at some time. This is partially caused by pressure of the pancreatic tumor on surrounding organs or nerves. Pain may also develop if the disease spreads outside of the pancreas to other parts of the body. The pain is most commonly felt in the upper abdomen and/or in the back. It may be experienced in many different ways (e.g., as discomfort, aching, a gnawing feeling, a sharp stabbing sensation, or cramping) and may be mild and intermittent or severe and continuous.

Many people are concerned about taking pain medication. Some people feel it is important to withstand pain as a sign of strength and that it is a part of having cancer that they have to accept. Some people are afraid of "masking" a problem and that if they treat the pain their doctor will not be able to follow their response to treatment. You should recognize that there is no benefit at all in having pain. Regardless of how mild the pain is, chronic pain can be very disabling. It affects your energy level, your appetite, your ability to sleep, your desire to be with friends and family, and your mood. You should tell your doctor or nurse about any discomfort that you have—no matter how mild it is. Try to describe it accurately so that they can decide on the best treatment for you and can monitor how effectively that treatment is working. When describing your discomfort, try to tell them about the following things: where you feel the pain; how severe the pain is (many doctors and nurses will ask you to rate the severity, e.g., using a scale of 0 to 10, with 0 being no pain at all and 10 being the worst pain that you can imagine);

There is no benefit at all in having pain.

what the pain feels like (e.g., sharp, achy, or gnawing); whether you have the pain all the time or only at certain times; what makes it worse and what makes it better; and how it affects your ability to sleep, your appetite, your activity, your desire to be with friends and family, and your mood.

Analgesics

medications to relieve pain.

Steroid

a category of medication with many different uses; most often used to reduce an inflammatory response.

There are many medications available for treating pain (called **analgesics**). Prescription medications are usually the most effective for treating pancreatic cancer pain. Narcotics are used most commonly. Some non-narcotic medications, including certain antidepressant, anticonvulsant, anti-inflammatory, and **steroid** medications, can help to relieve pain when used in combination with narcotics.

Pain medications come in many forms: tablets, liquids to swallow, liquids that are absorbed under the tongue, skin patches, and rectal suppositories. There are also solutions that can be given intravenously (into the vein) via a portable pump that is usually set to deliver a steady dose of medication into the blood stream with extra doses that you can deliver as needed. The pump is set up to allow "patient-controlled" medication administration with a limit to prevent overdose.

Pain medication for chronic pain works the most effectively when it is given "around the clock." This keeps a steady level of pain medication in your blood stream so that you don't have to experience pain. New long-acting medications are very helpful because they last for many hours or even days. To keep your pain controlled with these, you do not need to take medication as often as with the immediate-release short-acting forms; however, even with long-acting medication, most people also require an immediate-release pain medication for "breakthrough" pain, times when you experience discomfort during the day despite taking the long-acting medication around the clock. Be sure to ask your doctor or nurse for a prescription for an immediate-release pain medication with your long-acting medication. When using the immediate-release pain medication, take it as often as you need. If you wait too long between doses and the pain becomes severe, the medication will not work as quickly or as effectively. If you find that you need the immediate-release pain medication very frequently during the day or that it is not effective, ask your doctor about increasing the dose of the long-acting medication.

Some people are concerned about taking pain medication because of the side effects. Common side effects that people experience from pain medication include sleepiness, nausea, and constipation. Sleepiness generally passes after a few days; however, if this persists, you can ask your doctor or nurse to adjust the dose or add another medication to counteract the sleepiness. Nausea also commonly passes after a few days on pain medication, but if you have constant nausea, ask your doctor about trying a different pain medication or about taking an antinausea medication. Unfortunately, constipation from pain medications does not pass; however, taking a combination of a stool softener (e.g., Colace) and a laxative (e.g., Senekot, Lactulose, Miralax) on a regular basis can prevent this. Ask your doctor or nurse about which medications to take, what dose, and how often to take these. Increasing the amount of liquid that you drink during the day will also help reduce the likelihood of constipation. If you become dizzy or confused from the pain medication, tell your doctor or nurse. Switching the dose or type of medication usually resolves these problems.

Some people are concerned about taking pain medication because they are afraid of becoming addicted. Pain medication taken on a regular basis does cause tolerance. This is when your body physically adjusts to the level of medication in your blood stream. If you stop the medication suddenly, you can develop withdrawal symptoms. Tapering down the dose of medication gradually if you no longer need it, rather than stopping it suddenly, can prevent this. Your doctor or nurse will review with you exactly how to do this. Tolerance to the medication is not addiction, which is a desire or craving for the medication to feel high rather than to have your pain relieved. Research studies show that it is extremely rare for patients with cancer to develop addiction to pain medication.

It is extremely rare for patients with cancer to develop addiction to pain medication.

Some people are concerned about taking pain medication because they are afraid that if they take it for milder pain it won't work when they need it later for severe pain. Many pain medications, particularly narcotics, have no maximal dose that can be given. The dose can be increased indefinitely over time, and thus, you can be sure to get good pain relief if you need it at some point in the future no matter how severe your pain.

Many different types of pain medication are available, and what works for one person may not work as well for another. It may take some time to find the right medication, dose, and schedule to stop the pain. Be persistent in working with your doctor and nurse until you find a treatment that works for you. If you do not feel satisfied with the degree of relief that you are getting, ask about a referral to a pain specialist, who can also be found by calling the Cancer Information Service of the National Cancer Institute or the American Cancer Society.

73. Are there other treatments for pain that do not rely on medication?

Radiation therapy is effective in treating some types of cancer pain by shrinking a tumor that is pressing on surrounding organs or nerves. If you do not feel that your pain is adequately controlled with the medication that you are taking, ask your doctor if radiation therapy would be helpful in treating your pain; however, if cancer has spread throughout your body, radiation is unlikely to be helpful.

If pain is caused by pressure on a nerve, a nerve block (either a celiac axis or splanchic nerve block) can sometimes be performed. This involves injecting a local anesthetic or alcohol into or around the nerve near the point where the tumor is pressing. This blocks the spread of messages from the nerve up to the brain; thus, you will no longer be aware of the pressure. This may also be done surgically; the nerves are cut to relieve the pain. If you do not feel that your pain is controlled adequately with your current medication, ask your doctor if this would be helpful.

A variety of other strategies (e.g., distraction, relaxation, imagery, prayer, meditation, and acupuncture) may be helpful in treating pain; however, in pancreatic cancer, they are usually most effective if used in combination with pain medication. Specialists can perform these or train you to use these techniques to control your pain. Ask your doctor or nurse for a referral or contact the National Center for Complementary and Alternative Medicine.

For more information on how to manage pain, the National Cancer Institute has a booklet entitled "Pain Control: A Guide for People with Cancer and Their Families" that is available on the Internet (*oesi.nci.nih. gov/paincontrol/index.html*) or can be ordered by calling the Cancer Information Service.

Joy's Comment:

Two years after my surgery I had pain in my rectal area where the pancreatic cancer had "presented" itself. I had, for the second time, radiation and chemotherapy. The doctors said the pain should go away fairly quickly; when it didn't, they then said that sometimes it doesn't go away quickly! The pain did go away, miraculously, about 3 weeks after treatment ended.

74. I never feel hungry and am concerned about losing weight. What can I do to increase my appetite and maintain my weight?

Weight loss is a common problem for people with cancer. Having cancer changes your **metabolism**, which results in your needing many more calories each day than you usually eat. In addition, symptoms of the disease or side effects of treatment may make it difficult to eat or drink enough nutrients and fluids. You may have no desire for food or a feeling of being full after only a few bites of food. You may find that food tastes different or that symptoms such as nausea, gas, or con-

Metabolism

the physical and chemical processes required to maintain life.

stipation make it difficult to eat. Having pain, feeling tired, or experiencing emotional distress can also affect your appetite. In addition, changes in how your body digests or absorbs food may make it difficult for you to use the nutrients and fluids.

Taking in enough food and fluids is important in providing energy to your body and in helping you to handle treatment. For these reasons, if at all possible, try to maintain your usual weight or reduce the amount of weight that you are losing. You can do a number of things to improve your appetite and to help maintain your weight.

Medication may be helpful if you are having symptoms (e.g., mouth sores, nausea, vomiting, diarrhea, constipation, pain, or emotional distress) that affect your appetite. Ask your doctor for medication to relieve these symptoms. Also, following pancreatic surgery, many people do not secrete enough digestive enzymes needed for food to be digested and absorbed. This may cause changes in your stool and loss of weight (see Question 61). If you feel that this is happening to you, ask your doctor about taking pancreatic enzymes by mouth. In addition, there is a medication called Megace that may improve your appetite. Ask your doctor if this would be helpful for you.

It is also helpful to make changes in your diet to maximize the amount of nutrients that you take in each day:

• Eat small amounts of food and liquids at a time (rather than trying to eat three full meals a day, eat six or eight snacks throughout the day). Always have food nearby to nibble on.

- Select foods that are high in protein and calories. Foods that many people find easy to eat when they are not very hungry include eggs, cottage cheese, yogurt, peanut butter on crackers, sandwiches with turkey or tuna fish, baked or broiled chicken, fish, or beef, and soups.

- Add a variety of things to recipes to enhance the flavor of food and to add calories (e.g., butter, honey, jelly, sour cream, cheese, yogurt, cream, and evaporated milk). *Eating Hints for Cancer Patients*, published by the National Cancer Institute, provides many helpful recipes.

- Experiment with different foods and different seasonings to find those that taste the best to you. Some people find that red meat does not taste as flavorful while getting chemotherapy; chicken and fish may taste better.

- Limit the amount of liquids that you drink with your meals so that you don't fill up on the liquid.

- Have a limited amount of caffeinated beverages (e.g., coffee, tea, and many sodas), as these will cause dehydration.

- Have a limited amount of carbonated beverages, as they will make you feel full.

- Replace liquids with no nutritional benefit (such as water or soda) with liquids that provide nutrients (such as cream soups, shakes, and fruit smoothies).

- Try nutritional supplements that are available in your local drugstore. These may be canned drinks, powders to be mixed with water or milk, or puddings. Your doctor or nurse may recommend specific supplements for you. You can also use Carnation Instant Breakfast by blending it with milk and adding ice cream, yogurt, and/or fruit.

Other suggestions are as follows: (1) Rinse your mouth before eating. Moistening your mouth may enhance the taste of your food. (2) Ask your doctor or nurse if it is safe for you to have a glass of wine or beer or a cocktail before your meal. Many people find that alcohol stimulates their appetite. (3) Avoid eating alone. Having company can make eating more enjoyable, and we often eat more when eating with someone else.

It is common for family members and friends to recommend special diets, high-protein drinks, or supplemental megavitamins and **antioxidants**. These should not be taken without first speaking with your doctor or nurse because they may interfere with your treatment or may be dangerous.

Family members who have worked hard to prepare special foods may feel frustrated if you push it away after only a few bites. Avoid conflicts, but remind them that you are only able to eat what your appetite allows. Remember that eating should be pleasurable. The most important thing is to eat what you want when you want it. You may find it helpful to speak with a registered dietitian (certified by the American Dietetic Association) for guidance about what to eat. Ask your doctor or nurse for a referral to a nutritionist with expertise in working with people who have cancer.

75. Why do some people with cancer of the pancreas develop a yellowing of the skin?

One of the functions of the liver is to make bile, a fluid that aids in digestion and contains **bilirubin**, which gives bile a yellowish green color. Bile is stored in the

Antioxidants

chemical substances that may protect your cells against the effects of free radicals, which can cause cell damage.

Bilirubin

substance produced in the liver when the body breaks down hemoglobin, the molecule in red blood cells that carries oxygen; it is yellowish green in color and is eliminated in bile.

gallbladder; after eating, the gallbladder pushes the bile out through the bile duct into the intestine where it works to digest certain types of food.

When a mass develops in the pancreas, it may press on the bile duct, blocking the flow of bile. Bilirubin then builds up in the blood stream, lodges in the skin and eyes, and causes jaundice, a yellowing of the skin and eyes. Some of this excess bilirubin will be gotten rid of in the urine, causing it to become darker in color. Because the bilirubin is not able to pass into the intestine, the stools become lighter in color. Jaundice can also develop as a result of a tumor growing in the liver.

Sometimes jaundice can be treated. If the bile duct is blocked in a limited area, a small hollow tube can be inserted to open up the duct, relieving the blockage (see Question 21). However, if the jaundice cannot be treated, there are ways to make you comfortable.

Jaundice itself causes no pain; however, the skin may become very dry and itchy. Scratching may create breaks in the skin that could become infected; thus, preventing itching is important. Treating the dryness will help reduce the itching. When bathing, avoid very hot water and use only mild soaps. Apply skin lotions or creams after bathing and throughout the day as needed to moisturize the skin. If you still feel itchy, ask your doctor for a prescription for medication that will reduce the itching.

76. Why are my legs swollen? What can I do to minimize this?

People with cancer can develop swelling in their legs for the following reasons: (1) A lot of weight loss decreases the amount of protein in the blood, causing fluid to leak out of the blood vessels and accumulate in the tissues (e.g., the feet, ankles, and legs because gravity pulls the fluid downward). (2) Certain chemotherapy drugs (including gemcitabine on occasion) and other medications may cause fluid retention. This excess fluid may leak out of the blood vessels and lead to swelling. (3) A tumor in the abdomen or pelvis can put pressure on the lymph vessels and veins coming up from the legs. These vessels run throughout your body and carry fluid that normally collects in the tissues back into the bloodstream. If the vessels become blocked, they lose their ability to carry the fluid out of the tissues, leading to swelling. (4) Blood clots may form in the veins of the leg, blocking the flow of blood up from the legs. This usually occurs in only one leg. This is accompanied by swelling of the vein, usually causing redness, heat, and/or pain in the leg as well. This condition is known as **deep vein thrombosis**. Patients with cancer of the pancreas are particularly at risk for this problem and must be treated as soon as possible to prevent serious complications (see Question 77).

Deep vein thrombosis
presence of a blood clot in a deep vein.

Depending on the cause of swelling, there are a number of strategies to help reduce swelling and increase your comfort. Be sure your shoes, socks, and pants are not too tight. This may squeeze the vessels in your leg and increase the swelling. You may need to purchase shoes and socks that are bigger than your usual size. If you do not have a blood clot in your leg, you can also purchase special compression stockings at your drug store that will improve the ability of the vessels to return excess fluid from the legs; however, it is important that these fit correctly to avoid constriction and worsening of the problem. If you notice indented rings in the skin of your legs when you remove your socks or stockings, they are too tight. Walking may also be helpful because it causes tightening of your leg muscles, which supports the ability of the vessels to return excess fluid from the legs. Try to walk short distances often throughout the day; however, avoid standing in one place for long periods of time. Whenever sitting, keep your legs raised so that your feet are higher than your knees, which are higher than your hips. This way gravity will help pull the fluid out of your legs. Water pills or diuretics may be helpful if the swelling is from fluid retention; however, some people may become dehydrated from diuretics, and thus, they should only be taken if your doctor prescribes them. If the swelling is from fluid retention, reducing the amount of salt in your food may also be helpful.

77. What is deep vein thrombosis? How is it diagnosed and treated?

Patients with cancer of the pancreas are at risk for developing deep vein thrombosis. A blood clot forms in the vein of the leg, which blocks the flow of blood up from the leg, causing swelling. This is accompanied by inflammation of the vein, usually causing redness, heat, and/or pain in the leg as well. If left untreated, the blood clot will build up over time. It is possible that pieces of the blood clot will break off, travel to other parts of the body, and then block a blood vessel to one of your vital organs (e.g., the lung).

If your doctor suspects that the swelling may be from a blood clot, an ultrasound examination of your leg may be ordered. This simple test shows the veins in your legs and detects whether clots are present.

If the diagnosis is confirmed, treatment will be started immediately so as to prevent the blood from forming additional clots. This is called anticoagulation. Over time, the body will naturally break down the clot that has already developed. Initially, heparin is the most commonly used drug. It can be given by continuous intravenous infusion, requiring hospitalization for a number of days, or by an injection under the skin with a small needle several times a day. New low molecular weight heparin is increasingly being used. It provides several advantages: it can be given safely at home with only two injections a day; the dose can be determined more accurately than with other forms of heparin; and there is no need to have frequent blood tests to monitor its effects.

For most patients, an oral anticoagulant medication called warfarin (Coumadin) is also begun within a day or two of starting heparin; however, warfarin takes several days to a week to reach the right level in your blood. There is no standard dose of warfarin; the dose that you take will be determined by its effect on your blood. Two blood tests, the Prothrombin Time and the Internationalized Normal Ratio (INR), are used. Your doctor will adjust your dose of warfarin until the INR reaches a therapeutic level (between two and three). At that time, the heparin is usually stopped. You will continue on the warfarin for at least 6 months. If you have advanced pancreatic cancer, it is likely that you will have to stay on this medication for the rest of your life. Throughout that time, you will have to have periodic blood tests done (anywhere from twice a week to once a month) to confirm that your dose is correct. Adjustments in the dose are made as needed to keep the INR between two and three.

It is important that you take the exact dose of warfarin that is prescribed each night, as small changes in the dose can have very large effects on your blood. If you do not take enough warfarin, you may develop more blood clots, but if you take too much, you may develop bleeding. If you notice any signs of bleeding, contact your doctor or nurse immediately.

The metabolism of warfarin may be affected by certain foods, causing the warfarin to have either a greater or lesser effect at the same dose. Ask your pharmacist to give you a list of foods that interact with warfarin, and try to avoid these. In addition, warfarin can interact with a variety of medications. Always make sure to tell any doctor who prescribes you medication that you are taking this drug.

Always make sure to tell any doctor who prescribes you medication that you are taking this drug.

Occasionally patients with pancreatic cancer develop new or worsening blood clots despite being treated with an adequate dose of warfarin. In this circumstance, your doctor may choose to put you back on heparin on a long-term basis. An alternative treatment would be to put a special filter in the inferior vena cava, one of the large veins of your body, to prevent blood clots from traveling to the lung. If you have a filter, you do not need to take any anticoagulant medication.

PART SIX

Emotional and Social Concerns

How do I tell my family and friends that
I have cancer of the pancreas?

How do I tell my children/grandchildren
I have cancer?

More ...

78. How do I tell my family and friends that I have cancer of the pancreas?

For many people, having cancer is a lonely experience. Keeping your diagnosis a secret prevents others from being able to offer their help and support and will increase your loneliness. You may not be ready to share your thoughts and feelings right away, and thus, you might need to tell those who want you to talk before you are ready that you appreciate their concern but that you aren't ready to open up yet. Don't push them away; reassure them that you will speak with them when you are ready. When you are ready to talk about the diagnosis, decide what you want to share with others. When you do actually tell people about what is happening, you will probably find that being direct and honest is the easiest approach. Some people even find it helpful to rehearse what they will say.

Some friends or family members will be uncomfortable to hear about your diagnosis. They may pull away from you—not calling or visiting as they once did. This is probably because of their own fears about cancer or because they do not know what to say. If you don't care about keeping the relationship with this person, there is no reason to spend any time or energy trying to reach out; however, if you value this relationship, you may want to call and let this person know that you miss them. Tell them that you wish you could speak with them or see them more often, and ask if there is anything you can do to make it easier for them. This may break the ice and help them to feel more comfortable. Nevertheless, you will still find that some people will disappoint you; however, others will surprise you in their willingness to be helpful and supportive.

79. How do I tell my children/ grandchildren I have cancer?

It is a common reaction to try to protect children from the news that a family member has cancer for fear of upsetting them; however, children can always sense when something is wrong at home, and it is much better that they hear what is happening from you rather than by accidentally overhearing something or imagining something worse.

It is much better that they hear what is happening from you.

Children will cope best when they are informed. Set aside time to talk with them as soon as possible after you have been diagnosed, and be open and honest with them. You may want to include the following: the fact that you are sick and that you have cancer, the type of treatment that is planned, whether you will need to be in the hospital for a period of time, and the likely side effects of treatment and how they will affect how you look and what you will be able to do.

When speaking with children, select language that is age appropriate. It might be particularly helpful to practice what you want to say before you sit down with them.

After you have spoken with them, encourage the children to ask questions, and check to see that they understand what you have told them. You may need to break down the information and address only one or two topics at a time.

The children may ask if you will die, or they may ask for reassurance that you will get better. Respond to their questions as honestly as you can. Tell them that you are hoping that you will be okay and that the doctor is doing everything possible. If they ask you when

Emotional and Social Concerns

your treatment will be over, it is okay to tell them that you don't know. Reassure them that as things change, you will tell them about what is happening.

Describe how your disease and treatment will affect them. Explain who will take care of them if you will be in the hospital or if you will be coming home late from a doctor's visit or treatment. Explain how your disease and treatment will affect their usual routines and activities. Be sure to ask them if there is anything in particular that they are worried about. These two sources may help you to speak with children about cancer (including age-specific words to use in explaining the disease and treatment):

- *When a Parent is Sick: Helping Parents Explain Serious Illness to Children*, by Joan Hamilton, published by Pottersfield Press through Nimbus Publishing (ISBN 1–895–900–40–9; phone, 1–800-NIM-BUS–9 [1–800–646–2879]).
- *When Someone in Your Family has Cancer*, published by the National Cancer Institute, for young people who have a parent or other family member with cancer.

80. How can I better cope with having pancreatic cancer?

When confronted with any type of difficulty or stressful event, people tend to react and cope in their own ways. Some people turn away from what is happening and try to shut it out for a period of time, whereas others face things head on. Some are the most comfortable facing difficulties alone, whereas others prefer to have the support of family or friends. Sharing thoughts and feelings about the experience is common with some, yet others are more private and don't want to talk. Humor helps some people face their difficulties, whereas a more serious approach is used with others. Detailed information about what is happening is important for some patients, whereas for others, only a minimum of information is desired. Some people want to be actively involved in making all of the decisions, whereas others want their family or their doctor to make the decisions.

It is helpful for you to think about your preferences. How have you generally responded to difficulties in your life? Has this response worked for you in the past? Do you feel that it will be effective for facing your future challenges? If you feel comfortable with your method of coping and feel confident that it will continue to be helpful, there is no reason to change how you cope. In fact, you should explain to your family and friends and to your doctor and nurse about your best methods of coping. Thus, they can help to strengthen your ability to use these methods as you face the challenges that cancer poses.

Think about your preferences.

If you feel that your usual response isn't the most effective way of dealing with cancer, push yourself to try new coping methods. This is something that you may be able to do on your own or with help from your family and friends; however, many people may find it helpful to work with a professional therapist or counselor to learn new ways of coping with difficulties in their life (Question 89).

John's Comment:

With a lot of help physically, mentally, and spiritually, I coped with it. I think it started with my own attitude, which was "I will survive this." In fact, during my first meeting with the team at M. D. Anderson, I told them that while I accepted the risk of dying at any time, it was not *going to be from pancreatic cancer, so let's get going and fix this. But you must have a support team, starting with your immediate family and including other relatives and friends who are pulling for you and praying for you. I also had complete confidence in the medical team I was working with, and that is essential.*

Joy's Comment:

Initially, I was of the "don't really want to know" school because the news was all so negative. My surgeon routinely gives all his patients an antidepressant, which I took from surgery onward for about 3 months. I was never depressed, but this is also due to my incredible good fortune in being able to have surgery and that the cancer hadn't spread. Also, I looked upon it in many ways as a gift/sign to stop working and take joy in each day. A young woman I met later with pancreatic cancer said every day she asked herself "am I basking?" I try to do the same. Even though the cancer is recurring and I am undergoing continuing treatment, I still mostly feel this way. I'm definitely not "Polyanna," but going through all the treatment I have you see many, many people much worse off. There have been several times I've felt I was dying, and then have recovered. But the few times I have been "down" are nearly all related to food issues—finding food I want to eat and then trying to have it not flow right through me.

81. I feel so many different emotions throughout the day. How can I feel more in control?

When faced with a life-threatening illness, it is normal to react with many different emotions. You may find yourself denying the diagnosis at times and having difficulty acknowledging or accepting everything. You may feel angry that this is happening to you—angry at the medical establishment, angry at yourself, or even angry at God. You may feel worried about what treatment will be like and about your uncertain future. You may feel sad about the disruptions in your life, the loss of your independence, or the loss of all that you expected to be and experience in the future. Most people with cancer experience some or all of these feelings at one time or another. At certain times you can expect these feelings to be especially strong: when you are first told of the diagnosis, when you are faced with making decisions, just before you start treatment, if the cancer has returned or spread, or if an effective treatment for the cancer is no longer available. Do not be surprised if feelings that you thought had passed earlier come back to the surface at these times.

There are no right or wrong ways to feel. Trying to block or control your feelings may cause undue stress or suffering. Instead, allow yourself to experience your emotions, and try to understand and clarify what you are thinking and feeling. A number of ways of doing this are possible, and a combination of strategies may work best for you:

There are no right or wrong ways to feel.

- Mentally process your experience, and clarify in your mind what you are thinking and feeling.
- Write your thoughts and feelings in a journal.
- Talk about your thoughts and feelings with someone who you trust and feel support from (e.g., a close family member or friend, a professional counselor or therapist, or a religious leader or counselor). You may feel an immediate sense of relief once you have discussed your feelings aloud.
- Talk with other patients who are undergoing a similar experience and listen to how they describe their experiences.

Regardless of your approach, once you have recognized your thoughts and feelings, you will be better able to clarify what it is that you want and need. You can then direct your energy to getting these needs met, which will contribute to feeling more in control of the situation.

Other strategies can improve how you feel emotionally. Many people find that physical activity, even a brief walk, enhances their feeling of well-being. Others find that various relaxation techniques are helpful.

John's Comment:

Yes, I have periodic thoughts or fears about the cancer recurring—that is, I think, unavoidable. I counter them by looking at every day as a victory and being very thankful for the gift of life. For me, prayer is very helpful. Be positive—what do you have to lose by thinking that way?

82. Are there support groups where I can talk with other patients going through the same thing that I am?

Support groups can provide the opportunity to be with other cancer patients. You can share your thoughts and feelings with the group and hear how other people have reacted to and dealt with the same challenges that you are facing. This can be very helpful, as one of the most difficult parts of having cancer is feeling alone—feeling that no one really understands what you are going through.

Support groups are generally led by a health professional or a trained patient leader. They may be set up for people with only a particular kind of cancer or may be open to those with any type of cancer. They may be very structured or more social and informal. The groups may be very educationally focused, with speakers on different topics, or may provide interaction and sharing of people's individual experiences. Just the patients, just the families, or both may be allowed to participate. The group may meet for a defined period of time with a limited membership or may be open ended, allowing you to come and go as you like. Decide what would be most helpful to you when selecting a specific group; however, because pancreatic cancer is relatively uncommon, it is unlikely that you will find a support group of patients who have only this disease.

Increasing numbers of online support groups exist, and some of these are for patients with pancreatic cancer. Because many of these groups are not moderated by a professional and the information that you receive may not be accurate, you should discuss with your doctor the advice that you receive from an online support group.

You can find out about support groups that are near where you live or that are on the Internet in one of the following ways:

- Ask your doctor or nurse.
- Call the department of social work at your local hospital.
- Contact Cancer Care, the American Cancer Society, or the Cancer Information Service of the National Cancer Institute.
- Get in touch with Gilda's Club (*www.gildasclub.org* or 1–917–305–1200).
- Contact the Wellness Community (www.*wellness-community.org* or 1–888–793-WELL).

- Look up the Association of Cancer Online Resources (*www.acor.org*).
- Go to OncoChat (*www.oncochat.org*).

83. My body seems different now that I have cancer. I don't feel as attractive as I once did. What can I do to feel better about myself?

You are likely to be aware of changes in your body after you have been diagnosed with cancer. Some things you can see (e.g., scars from surgery, drainage tubes, venous catheters, loss of hair, or a change in your weight); however, others may not be visible at all—just a feeling that your body is different and knowing that things inside are not the way they used to be. In addition, you may not be able to do some of the things that you used to do at work or at home or for enjoyment. These things may affect how you see yourself as a person or how attractive you feel as a man or woman.

Although it may not be possible to reverse these physical changes, you can do some things to feel better about how you look. You may want to select some new clothes or have some favorite clothes altered to fit better if you have lost weight. Some women find that using makeup, having a manicure or pedicure, and wearing scarves helps them feel better about how they look. In addition, the American Cancer Society and the Cosmetic, Toiletry, and Fragrance Association sponsor a free program ("Look Good, Feel Better") that is dedicated to helping women with cancer feel better about their appearance. They teach beauty techniques that help to restore your appearance and improve your self-image. You can check on their Internet site (*www.lookgoodfeelbetter.org*) to see whether it is available in your area, or you can call the American Cancer Society.

It is also helpful to think about what makes you who you are. Is it the way you look? Is it what you do? Is it what you have accomplished in the past? Is it your relationships with other people? Is it who you are as an individual—those intangible things in your mind, your heart, and your soul? While recognizing that some things have changed since your diagnosis with cancer, you should stay connected with those other things that make you who you are. Think about the accomplishments of your life. Plan time to be with people you enjoy. Continue to involve yourself in the things that give you intellectual satisfaction. Express your thoughts and feelings with those you trust and care about. Maintain your relatedness with whatever spirituality you feel connected to. All of these things will enhance your feelings about yourself.

84. I don't feel the desire to be sexually intimate with my partner the way I used to. What can I do to maintain my relationship with him or her?

Physical intimacy is one aspect of a loving relationship. It gives us personal pleasure and creates a feeling of closeness to our partner. Sexual intercourse is one way of being physically intimate; however, pain, fatigue, emotional distress, or the side effects of treatment may affect your desire for or ability to enjoy sex.

123

If you would like to continue having sexual intercourse with your partner, consider strategies that will make it more pleasurable for you. Take medication that has been prescribed for any bothersome symptoms. Select a time of day when you usually have more energy and when you know that you will have privacy. Experiment with different positions that might be more comfortable or less tiring. Of course, be sure to always use a safe method of birth control if there is a risk of pregnancy.

It is important to remember that there are many other ways of maintaining a physically intimate relationship with your partner without having intercourse. Cuddling, hugging, touching, rubbing, and holding hands can give pleasure. It is also important to talk with your partner about your physical relationship, your fears and concerns, and your hopes and desires. Talking together about these things will create a feeling of intimacy between you and your partner and will help each of you know the other's wants and needs so that you can experience pleasure being together.

It is also important to discuss your concerns with and ask questions of your doctor and nurse. They can explain how your disease and treatment may affect your sexuality. Sex therapists can provide counseling. You can get a referral from your doctor or nurse, from the Cancer Information Service of the National Cancer Institute, or from the American Association of Sex Educators, Counselors, and Therapists (*www.aasect*). In addition, the American Cancer Society has two excellent books that can be helpful: *Sexuality and Cancer: For the Woman Who Has Cancer, and Her Partner* and *Sexuality and Cancer: For the Man Who Has Cancer, and His Partner*.

85. Should I work during my treatment?

Some people feel quite well during their pancreatic cancer treatment and wish to continue working, either full-time or part-time; however, others do not. Thus, they must adjust their hours of work or the specific tasks that they do at work. Tell your doctor or nurse about the type and number of hours of work that you do. Ask them how they expect you to feel during treatment and what they recommend in regard to your continuing to work. If you are going to continue work, see Question 86 on things to consider when you tell your supervisor and coworkers about your illness. If you are unable to work or must switch to part-time work, speak with someone in the human resources department about your options. Find out about your disability benefits. Be aware that the Family and Medical Leave Act allows eligible employees up to a total of 12 weeks of unpaid leave during any 12-month period. For information about this, contact the human resources department where you work or the United States Department of Labor (*www.dol.gov/dol/esa/fmla.htm*).

Find out about your disability benefits.

86. Should I tell my supervisor and coworkers about my diagnosis?

You may be concerned about telling your supervisor or coworkers about the cancer diagnosis. Also, it is common to feel that cancer is a private matter; you may not want others to know, or you may not be sure how much to tell about your diagnosis or treatment. You may even be afraid that you will be treated differently, that you will be discriminated against, or that you may lose your job.

The Americans with Disabilities Act protects you from discrimination at work and requires that employers make reasonable adjustments as long as you can perform the essential functions of the job. Employers, however, unfortunately do not always respond the way that we hope that they will or that the law requires. You may find that your supervisor believes that you will not be able to perform as well on the job, and you may lose the opportunity to work on certain projects or even to be promoted. Your coworkers may be uncomfortable hearing about your diagnosis and may pull away from you—not talking as they once did. This is probably because of their own fears and anxieties about cancer or because they do not know what to say. Some coworkers may even worry that they will have to do more work because of your illness, which may make them resentful.

If you need accommodations in the type of work that you do or in the hours that you work, prepare ahead for this conversation and then speak with your supervisor about the situation. First, determine how you can get the most important parts of your job done. Then determine how you need to alter the hours you work to balance getting the job done with taking care of your medical needs. Being open with your supervisor at the beginning can be extremely helpful because they can guide you in obtaining information about your rights and benefits and can work with you to make the necessary adjustments. If you find it difficult to speak directly with your supervisor about this, talk with someone in the human resources department. If you have a conflict with your supervisor and the human resources department is not able to help, you may need to contact an attorney for guidance. For more information about the Americans with Disabilities Act and how it applies to you, contact the United States Department of Justice (*www.usdoj.gov/crt/ada/ada-hom1.htm* or 1–800–514–0301) or the United States Equal Employment Opportunity Commission (*www.eeoc.gov/* or 1–202–663–4900).

87. How do we manage the financial burdens that cancer places on our family?

The financial burdens related to diagnosing and treating cancer are enormous. It will be helpful at the beginning of your illness to choose a main person to deal with all of the financial issues. You may want to manage this yourself, but be aware that many people find that while dealing with the details of their disease and treatment they are not able to focus on the many financial issues that must be addressed. It will be helpful if a family member or friend can take over this responsibility for you. A number of steps can be taken to help manage this responsibility.

Review your healthcare benefits thoroughly to determine what help is available. Many policies are confusing; if you do not understand your benefits, speak with someone in your human resources department or contact the insurance company directly. You may want to ask the following specific questions:

- Can any doctor treat you, or must you use someone outlined in your plan?
- How much more will you have to pay if you use a doctor outside of your plan ("out of network")?

- Do you have coverage for a second opinion?
- Do you need authorization before having particular diagnostic tests or treatments? What is the process for obtaining this?
- Does the plan cover care at only certain hospitals?
- Does the plan provide home care with only certain agencies?
- What coverage do you have for prescription medications?

A financial counselor where you will be receiving treatment can help to determine the estimated costs of care. Work with them to calculate what you will have to pay out of pocket based on the insurance coverage that you have. If you are not able to pay this, discuss how you can work out a realistic payment plan.

If you have difficulty paying for care, meet with a social worker to find out what financial assistance is available. You may be entitled to government or charitable assistances, and the American Cancer Society and Cancer Care may also be able to provide financial assistance.

The cost of prescription medications can be significant, and thus, many pharmaceutical companies have assistance programs to provide medication at a reduced cost. To find out about financial assistance available for particular medications, ask your nurse or social worker for information. Cancer Care has a web site (*www.cancercare.org/hhrd/drug_assistance.asp*) that lists pharmaceutical companies with assistance programs.

Transportation also causes the financial costs to increase quickly. If you need assistance with transportation, speak with a social worker to get information about transportation services in your region. Cancer Care and the American Cancer Society can also provide information and may be able to offer limited financial assistance for transportation.

Throughout your treatment, track all of the financial costs that you have incurred because of this illness. Speak with your accountant when you are first diagnosed for information on what is tax deductible and what records he or she may want you to keep. For most people, medical costs not covered by insurance are tax deductible. These include your annual deductible costs, co-pays (the fees you pay up front for specific services), and coinsurance (the part of the bill your insurance company doesn't cover). Keep copies of all bills and claim forms. The money that you pay toward your health insurance policy is tax deductible. Other costs (e.g., prescription medications or the mileage for trips to appointments) may also be tax deductible. Keep receipts for all of these out-of-pocket expenses.

88. My emotions are often overwhelming, and I feel upset much of the time. How do I know whether I should seek professional help?

As described in Question 81, it is normal to react with many different emotions after being diagnosed with cancer; however, you should differentiate normal emotional reactions from those that cause significant stress or suffering. Some signs that you are in distress include the following:

- You are having so much difficulty accepting the reality of what is happening to you that you can't make decisions about your care.
- You are so angry that you aren't able to feel trust in your healthcare providers.
- You are so worried and anxious that you find it difficult to understand and absorb the information that you are getting, you are having difficulty making decisions, or you are having difficulty solving everyday problems.
- Your feel severe uncontrolled anxiety much of the time, with a constant feeling that something dreadful is going to happen. This may be accompanied by feeling nervous, shaky, or jittery; sweating; feeling tightness in your chest or stomach; or feeling that your heart is racing.
- You are sad and tearful throughout most of the day.
- You become depressed and lose interest or pleasure in those aspects of your life that you have previously enjoyed. Feelings of despair or hopelessness or problems with energy, sleep, appetite, or concentration may accompany this.
- You find yourself unable to communicate as you usually do with your family or friends.

Addressing emotional distress is as important as attending to any of your physical symptoms.

If you are experiencing any of these signs continuously for more than 2 weeks or if your feelings become very upsetting or interfere with your daily life, discuss these symptoms with your doctor or nurse. Addressing emotional distress is as important as attending to any of your physical symptoms. Ask your doctor or nurse about obtaining help from a mental health professional. Seeking this kind of treatment is not a sign of weakness and in fact can enhance your ability to cope. This is particularly true if you have had anxiety or depression in the past. Treatment can involve thera-peutic counseling, medication, and a variety of tech-niques using your body and mind (Question 57). Question 89 discusses how to find professional help.

89. Where can I get professional help in dealing with my emotional concerns or to improve my ability to cope with having cancer?

Many ways are available for getting professional help in dealing with your emotions and improving your ability to cope with having cancer. (1) Mental health professionals include psychiatrists, psychologists, social workers, and psychiatric nurses. They are all licensed or certified in their specialty and can provide counsel-ing. Psychiatrists and some psychiatric nurses can pre-scribe medication. (2) Religious leaders and counselors or hospital chaplains can help you to find strength and support in the spiritual dimension of your life.

You can get a referral to one of these professionals by asking your doctor or nurse; contacting your hospital's department of social work, department of psychiatry, or chaplaincy service; contacting Cancer Care, the American Cancer Society, or the Cancer Information Service of the National Cancer Institute; and speaking with the religious leader at your local house of worship.

FOR FAMILY AND FRIENDS
90. How can I help?

It is difficult to know the best way to help someone who has been diagnosed with cancer. No answer to this question is right for everyone. You have to match what you are able and would like to do with the specific things that are needed.

You may find it easiest to start with concrete things. A general offer of "let me know if I can help with anything" may not actually be the best approach and may create a burden, as the person must think about what he or she needs and then ask you for help. Instead, try to anticipate what he or she will need and make specific offers. Plan these for days when you know that the person may need more help than usual (e.g., days of doctor's visits or treatment or when he or she is feeling particularly ill or tired). The possibilities are unlimited, but examples of things that you might offer include driving the patient to a doctor's visit or treatment, dropping off a dinner for the family, spending a morning cleaning the house, laundering the family clothes, shopping for food and needed household items, inviting his or her children for a sleepover, and arranging to pick up or meet the patient's children after school.

You can also offer help by being available. Would the person appreciate company because he or she lives alone or because the rest of the family is working or at school? Offer to visit and bring lunch, to accompany the person for a walk, to bring a video that you can both watch, to go shopping together, or to have the patient come spend the weekend with you. Again, the possibilities are unlimited. The key is to match what you are able and would like to do with the specific things that he or she enjoys. One word of caution, however—this person may not have the energy to participate in many of the things that you used to do together. Consider how the patient is feeling at the time and don't create unrealistic expectations for him or her. You may need to plan short visits, and your time together should be pleasurable regardless of what you do or how long you spend together.

Joy's Comment:

For me, the best gift anyone could give me was/is home-cooked food because I don't enjoy cooking and food is always an issue.

91. What is the right thing to say?

It is natural to feel unsure of the right things to say when someone you care about has been diagnosed with cancer, is undergoing difficult treatment, or is perhaps facing the end of his or her life. You may feel uncomfortable asking the person how he or she is doing because you are unsure of the response. You may worry that if you say the wrong thing, you will hurt him or her, or that if you talk about your own sadness, or even cry, the person will be upset. Because of your own discomfort, you may try to withdraw from the situation, distancing yourself from the person, calling less often, and putting off visits. This can result in leaving the person feeling alone at a time when he or she needs your presence more than ever before.

It is natural to feel unsure of the right things to say.

There is no script you can follow as a guide in knowing what to say. In fact, if you make assumptions about what the person is thinking or feeling, you may unintentionally say things that will be upsetting. The best way to start is by listening. Let the person know that if he or she would like to talk about their illness you would like to listen. At the same time, remember that not everyone communicates in the same way. Some

The best way to start is by listening.

Emotional and Social Concerns

people are very open and want to share all their thoughts and feelings. Others are more private and prefer not to talk about these things. Even for those who are generally more communicative, there may be times that he or she may feel like talking and other times when he or she doesn't. You should let the person know that you are available to listen and should let them control when and how much they choose to share. This is a great gift that you can give.

However, listening to things that are painful or being with someone who is emotionally upset or crying may be uncomfortable. You may want to change the subject or even offer reassurances that everything will be okay, even if that may not necessarily be true. Although this may help in dealing with your own discomfort as the listener, it does not help the person speaking. In addition, it may give the message that you do not really want to hear what he or she has to say. Try to overcome your own discomfort and remain to hear what he or she is saying. It is okay to tell the person that this is difficult for you and that you are not sure how to respond to what is being said.

You also may want to speak to the person who is ill about thoughts or feelings that you are having. You may want to tell him or her about your love and concern or of your own sadness or feelings of helplessness. You may want to try to resolve previous conflicts. You may want to talk with him or her about your own worries and concerns related to the illness. We often leave a great deal unsaid in an attempt to protect those we love. Yet in fact, it is the unsaid things that are often the most important to say.

92. At times I feel overwhelmed by the responsibility of caring for this person. Do other people experience similar feelings?

When someone is diagnosed with pancreatic cancer, numerous stresses and demands are placed on family and friends. The patient's age, the role that they play in the family, how advanced the disease is, the type of treatment they are getting, the symptoms that they are experiencing, how physically disabled they are, and how they are emotionally responding to their illness—all of these factors will affect the stresses placed on the family. Regardless of the individual situation, there are several sources of stress for those who are providing care.

One demand placed on caregivers is the need to provide physical care to the person who is ill. The past 20 years have brought many changes in healthcare. One of the most significant is that people who were previously cared for in the hospital are now cared for at home. This places the responsibility of providing physical care on family and friends. This includes ensuring that the person is comfortable; administering medications; managing equipment and supplies; observing for relevant signs or symptoms; knowing when to call the doctor or nurse; and if the person is very ill, helping with bathing, dressing, feeding, moving, and walking. If the person has advanced disease, these demands will increase as the person gets sicker.

Another demand placed on caregivers is the need to address the nonmedical aspects of care, including scheduling and coordinating appointments, providing transportation, obtaining medications, running errands, supervising others who are providing care, as well as handling medical bills and other financial matters. In addition, numerous decisions will need to be made every day, and the need to solve problems will regularly arise.

Making this even more difficult is the fact that when you become a caregiver your usual day-to-day responsibilities don't just go away, and you may also have to take on those responsibilities previously handled by the person who is now ill. If your previous relationship with the patient has been difficult, you may have mixed feelings about the fact that you now need to provide this person's care.

The stresses and demands placed on you as a caregiver can lead you to feel overwhelmed at times. You may become exhausted or even physically ill. In addition, you may find yourself experiencing a variety of difficult emotions: anger, guilt, fear, and sadness. You must find ways of caring for yourself—attending to your physical and emotional needs. Only then can you effectively attend to the needs of the person who is ill and make this experience meaningful.

You must find ways of caring for yourself— attending to your physical and emotional needs.

93. How can I get help so that I can provide support and care to this person without being overwhelmed?

The physical and emotional demands of care giving are significant. The first step to getting help is acknowledging how this is affecting you and identifying which demands are the greatest. Are you having difficulty finding enough time needed for care—visiting in the hospital, accompanying the person to doctor's visits or treatments, having to do more at home, or needing to take time off of work? Are you having difficulty with the finances: inadequate medical insurance for doctor's visits and treatments, expensive medication, costs of travel, costs of missed work time, costs of extra services (e.g., extra babysitting)? Are you having difficulty with the physical burdens of providing care if the person is weak and debilitated—needing to assist with walking or lifting, needing to bathe and feed, needing to administer medications, perhaps needing to move in with them for a period of time? Are you having difficulty with the overall responsibility of managing care when you don't feel that you have adequate knowledge or skills to do this effectively?

Several approaches are available to help you manage the demands of caregiving. Most important is that you have the necessary information to feel capable of providing care. Schedule time to speak with the person's doctor or nurse in the office or over the phone to review the plan of care and to discuss your concerns. Some specific questions that you may want to ask include the following:

- What is the goal of treatment?
- What do you expect will be the outcome of the treatment?
- What side effects may occur from the treatment?
- How can the side effects be managed?
- What medications have been prescribed? What are they for? What dose should be given and at what times of the day?
- What are reasons I should call your office?

Ask whether they have any written material that reinforces this information.

To manage the many things that must be done each day, divide the work. Identify who among family members and friends is able and willing to do various parts of the work; however, it is important to recognize that characteristics of people at times of stress don't generally change from those that they usually have. Instead, they tend to become more exaggerated; thus, families that generally work well together at times of stress will work well together in this situation, and families in which there is a previous history of disagreement may find it difficult to overcome patterns of conflict. Furthermore, each member of the family will have a different idea about what they can manage— one that may not match your own expectations. Based on each person's ability and willingness, assign a schedule for each person to do the various tasks.

If you need more assistance at home than family or friends can provide, ask your doctor or nurse to refer you to a social worker, who can review homecare services that are available. These services include having a registered nurse to make visits (e.g., changing a dressing and giving an injection), home health aides to assist with personal care (e.g., bathing or being present in the home to assist the person during hours that you're not available), and homemakers to assist with tasks at home (e.g., cooking, cleaning, and laundry). You will need to verify what services are covered with the person's health insurance company. If there is no coverage for help at home, consider whether you or other members of the family have the financial resources to pay for these services.

Other resources may be helpful in providing support to you as a caregiver. Educational programs designed specifically for caregivers of people with cancer may be available in your community. You can find out about these through the American Cancer Society, the Cancer Information Service of the National Cancer Institute, Cancer Care, or the department of social work at your local hospital. Three particularly good resources are as follows:

- The National Family Caregivers Association offers education and support to family caregivers (*www. nfcacares.org* or 1–800–896–3650).
- *Caregiving: A Step-By-Step Resource for Caring for the Person with Cancer at Home* is published by the American Cancer Society.
- *Caring for the Caregiver* is an audio program that was developed by the National Coalition for Cancer Survivorship, the Oncology Nursing Society, and the Association of Oncology Social Work (*www. cansearch.org/programs/Caregiver.PDF*).

The key to being able to provide care for someone else is to care for your own needs. Combat isolation by reaching out to people who can support you; spend time with them and talk about how things are going. Schedule time for yourself to do things that you enjoy (e.g., taking a walk, listening to music, or reading a book). Don't try to do everything yourself; divide the work and let others help.

The key to being able to provide care for someone else is to care for your own needs.

Caregiving is stressful and has many demands. It can be seen as a burden or as an opportunity. In caring for another person, you may learn of inner strengths that you never knew you had, and you may find that you are more competent and capable than you had previously realized. In caring for another person, you may feel spiritually enriched, and family and friends can come together with a renewed sense of purpose and connection. You also have the opportunity to express your love for that person in the most intimate way imaginable.

CHANGES IN TREATMENT

94. I have completed treatment and my doctor tells me that there is currently no evidence of cancer. What comes next?

Completing treatment for pancreatic cancer brings its own set of challenges. Among these are adjusting to changes in your body that may require you to eat differently or take new medications, recovering strength after treatment, resuming your usual activities, returning to work, and explaining your illness to friends and colleagues. Each of these presents a new hurdle to overcome. It is important to give yourself time and to remember to draw on your usual methods of coping as well as those that are newly learned as you transition into feeling "normal" again (Question 80).

Despite the fact that your treatment is over, you will probably find it difficult at times to balance the hopefulness that the disease will not come back with the knowledge that the future is always uncertain. You must maintain a schedule of regular follow-up visits with your doctor and have blood tests and scans periodically to evaluate how you are doing. The days immediately before your doctor's appointments and the days waiting for the results of diagnostic tests are often filled with anxiety and worry.

Three resources might be particularly helpful as you adjust to your life as a cancer survivor:

- *Facing Forward, A Guide for Cancer Survivors*, published by the National Cancer Institute, describes the experiences of other survivors, provides practical suggestions on specific topics, and lists resources for more detailed information.
- The Cancer Survivor's Network of the American Cancer Center (*www.acscsn.org*) offers recorded discussions on particular issues and provides an opportunity to interact with other survivors.
- The National Coalition for Cancer Survivorship (*www.cansearch.org*) is an advocacy organization for cancer survivors. They also have an audio program teaching skills of survivorship (*www.cansearch.org/programs/Caregiver.PDF*).

Despite the fears and uncertainties that lie ahead, some people find that having been diagnosed with cancer provides them with the opportunity to think about their lives in new ways. The experience enriches and strengthens relationships, and sometimes people choose to shift their priorities, ensuring they are spending their time doing the most important things.

95. How does my doctor evaluate if my treatment is working? What if my treatment doesn't work?

While you are undergoing treatment, you will be seeing your doctor regularly so that he or she can see how you are tolerating the treatment, if you are having side effects, and if so, how severe they are. The doctor may make adjustments in your treatment dose or schedule based on the side effects. The second reason for these visits is to see how your cancer is responding to the treatment. If you have had the cancer removed, the doctor will want to be sure that the cancer has not reappeared. If the cancer could not be removed, the doctor will want to be sure that it is not growing or metastasizing (spreading to other areas). To assist in evaluating the response of the tumor, your doctor will order CT scans or MRIs on a regular basis, generally every 3 to 4 months.

Recurrence after pancreatic cancer has been surgically removed indicates that tiny cancer cells that could not be seen during surgery were left behind. Over time, these cells may divide and grow to form another tumor. If you are not receiving treatment at the time that you develop a recurrence, your doctor may recommend that you begin treatment with chemotherapy, radiation therapy, or a combination of both. If you develop a recurrence or if the tumor progresses or metastasizes while you are on treatment, the cancer cells have become resistant to the treatment that you are getting. If that happens, your doctor will likely recommend discontinuing your current treatment and will discuss other options with you.

If your energy level is good, your weight is fairly stable, and you are able to be up and around most of the day, it is more likely you will have a good response to active treatment; thus, your doctor may recommend a new type of treatment. The goal of this treatment would be to control any further growth of the tumor and to prolong your life as much as possible.

Hearing that your cancer has recurred after it was removed or that it has grown while you have been on treatment is obviously very upsetting. You may find yourself again experiencing many of the feelings that you had when you were first diagnosed—anger, sadness, worry, or even difficulty accepting the reality of what the doctor is saying. You may feel frightened that you will develop new physical symptoms, feel concerned about family and friends, be worried about the financial implications for your family, and may feel spiritually upset or have existential concerns. Questions 80 and 81 suggest how to deal with these emotions and concerns.

Getting accurate information from your doctor will be particularly important as you consider the next step. Some people find it helpful to have their doctor fully explain the details of their illness and their prognosis. Others prefer not to hear the details and to focus on the plan. Decide what you want to know, and communicate this to your family and doctor (see Question 80).

If you have been hoping for cure, hearing that your disease has recurred or grown will challenge the way that you have been thinking about your illness. It will require that you rethink your goals for treatment and reconsider what is most important to you knowing that you cannot be cured. Tell your family and your doctor and nurse about your concerns and your goals. A resource that may be helpful during this time is *When Cancer Recurs*, published by the National Cancer Institute.

96. My doctor has told me that I should discontinue active treatment because my disease is now advanced and can no longer be controlled. What does this mean?

If your tumor gets worse or metastasizes while you are on treatment, this indicates that the cancer cells have become resistant to the treatment you are getting. If that happens, your doctor will recommend discontinuing your current treatment. If you have already received many different types of treatment, your energy level is poor, you have lost a great deal of weight, and you are spending most of the day in bed, it is unlikely that active treatment will be effective for you.

Your life is not yet over.

You may feel very upset that your cancer can no longer be controlled and that you are now facing the end of your life. The sense of sadness and hopelessness may be overwhelming at times. It is important to remember that your life is not yet over and that by living one day at a time you can make each day a good one. Plan ahead; think about what is important to you, and do something that you enjoy every day. Plan special visits with family and friends. Attend religious services. Go out, if you feel up to it. Visit a special place where you have fond memories. Be with people you care about. A resource that may be helpful to you at this time is *Living with Advanced Disease*, published by the National Cancer Institute.

PREPARING FOR THE END OF LIFE

97. What is hospice? How can I find a hospice if I need one?

Hospice is a philosophy of care that addresses medical, physical, emotional, social, and spiritual needs to ensure quality of life for people who are at the end of their life. The focus is on palliative care—ensuring that you are comfortable, free of pain, and without troubling symptoms.

Hospice care is often provided at home, with family members providing most of your physical care. A team of hospice specialists works together to ensure that your needs are met and that your family has the support that they need for your care. Doctors are available to prescribe medical care and to ensure control of pain and other symptoms. Registered nurses will monitor how you are feeling and how your family is coping, and they will teach your family how to care for you. Social workers provide emotional support. Clergy provide spiritual support. Home health aides can assist in caring for physical needs (e.g., bathing), and volunteers offer their companionship. Hospice also provides all of the medical equipment, supplies, or medications that you would need. In addition, a nurse is on call 7 days a week, 24 hours a day to answer questions and to address problems that may arise at home. Hospice care can also be provided in an inpatient setting, either at a freestanding hospice facility, a nursing home, or a hospital. Additional information on hospice is available at National Hospice Foundation (*www.hospiceinfo.org* or 1–800–338–8619) or Hospice Net (*www. hospicenet.org*).

To be eligible for hospice, you must have a life-threatening illness, not be receiving curative treatment, and have a life expectancy of 6 months or less. Your doctor may recommend hospice care for you if he or she feels that chemotherapy or radiation therapy is no longer able to control your cancer. If you receive hospice care, your own doctor may be able to provide your medical care, or he or she may recommend that the hospice doctor, specially trained in palliative care, should take over. Your doctor, nurse, or social worker may recommend a particular hospice program to you, or you may be able to get a referral through your health insurance plan. In fact, some plans work only with particular hospices, and thus, you should contact them to clarify your hospice benefits. If you want to find out what hospices are available in your community, you can search for a local hospice through the National Hospice and Palliative Care Organization at their Internet site (*www.nhpco.org*) or by calling 1–800–658–8898.

98. What are advance directives? How can I be sure my wishes are known?

Advance directives are legal documents that describe what type of medical care you want to receive if you become unable to make decisions or speak for yourself. Although the specific laws and terminology for advance directives vary from state to state, two basic types of advance directives exist: a living will and a healthcare proxy.

A living will states specific instructions regarding your healthcare, particularly regarding measures that would lengthen your life. The document outlines those medical interventions that you want to have performed and those that you want to have withheld in a variety of circumstances.

You may want to specify a number of medical interventions in a living will. If you were to lose the ability to eat and drink, what would your wishes be regarding receiving nutrition through a feeding tube or intravenous fluids? If your heart were to stop beating or if you were to stop breathing, what are your wishes regarding resuscitation (e.g., performing cardiopulmonary resuscitation, putting a tube down your throat and connecting it to a breathing machine, or shocking your heart)?

When making these decisions, it is helpful to distinguish between the types of problems that could occur. If the problem is treatable and reversible, you may want all medical measures taken to resuscitate and support you. If the problem results from progressive cancer that can no longer be controlled, you may not want any extraordinary measures taken to resuscitate you or prolong your life. In that situation, some people want to sign a "do not resuscitate" order to ensure that none of these measures are taken. Making these decisions is very difficult, and there is no correct decision. You need to think about what you want for yourself, and these documents provide the opportunity for you to express this so that people can act on your decisions.

There are two limitations to a living will. First, not all states recognize a living will. Second, it is impossible to imagine all of the possible circumstances that might occur with your health. Decisions may need to be made that you have not thought to specify in writing.

Healthcare proxy

a health care surrogate, a medical proxy, or a medical power of attorney; a person authorized to make health care decisions for you if you are not able to

This problem can be avoided by designating a **health-care proxy** (also called a health care surrogate, a medical proxy, or a medical power of attorney), who is authorized to make healthcare decisions for you if you are unable. They can decide which medical interventions should be performed and which should be withheld. Although the terminology varies from state to state, a healthcare proxy is recognized in all states.

A healthcare proxy should be someone you trust and someone who will make decisions based on your desires—not on what he or she wants for you or on what he or she would want if they were in your position. You can choose a family member or a friend as your healthcare proxy. Talk with the person about what you would want in a variety of circumstances. Talk about the issues described previously here in regard to resuscitation and life-prolonging measures such as artificial nutrition and intravenous fluid. Be as specific as you are able. Then confirm with the person that he or she will honor your wishes and that he or she is willing to speak for you. You can change your healthcare proxy and your decisions about what you want done at any time.

It is helpful to let your family and friends know whom you have selected as your healthcare proxy so that conflict will be minimized and so that everyone can support this person in making the decisions. If you have completed a living will, it is important to share this with them as well. It is also important to tell all of your doctors and your medical team about your wishes. They should have copies of any advance directive documents that you have signed.

Having a discussion about what you would want if you were unable to make decisions for yourself is difficult for most people. Sometimes the person who is ill wants to bring it up but is afraid the family will be troubled by the conversation. Sometimes the family wants to bring it up but is afraid it will upset the patient. It is always better to talk about these things when you are feeling fairly well and when no forthcoming crisis is looming. This way you will be able to think calmly and to communicate clearly with each other about what you want.

The discussion can be started in several ways. You could say this: "I want to be sure that if I were to become sicker you would know what I want done." A family member could begin by saying this: "If you were to become sicker and couldn't tell me what kind of care you wanted, I wouldn't know what to do. Can we talk about this?" You may find that your family does not agree with the decisions that you have made. In this situation, you should have an advance directive to ensure that your wishes are honored.

You can obtain state-specific advance directive documents from your lawyer, your doctor, or your local hospital. The Partnership for Caring—a nonprofit organization whose mission is to improve how people die—also provides state-specific documents. In addition, they provide information on end-of-life issues and offer a national crisis and information hotline dealing with these issues (*www.partnershipforcaring. org/Advance/index.html* or 1–800–989–9455).

99. How do I plan for the possibility that I may die? How do I prepare my family and myself?

The reality of death is something we all must face; however, we generally don't think about our own death until we see it as an immediate threat—either by hearing about someone we know who has died or by being diagnosed ourselves with a life-threatening disease such as cancer. Regardless of how difficult and painful it may be to face the reality of your own death and the possibility of a premature death, doing so provides you with the opportunity to plan ahead.

Ideally, planning for death should be done when you are feeling well.

Ideally, planning for death should be done when you are feeling well, early in the course of your disease, when there is no actual threat of death. You can then take the time to thoughtfully make decisions about what you want. Planning for death is not giving up; instead, it creates the opportunity for you to shape how your life will end, whenever that occurs, whether from this disease or from some other cause. It also allows you to make arrangements for those you will leave behind. There are many specific ways in which you can plan.

As much as possible, plan for the financial issues that will arise for your family after you die. Work with an attorney to write a will, specifying what is to become of your property. If you have children or adults who are financially dependent on you, calculate what assets they will have, what income they can expect, and what expenses they will have. It may be helpful to meet with an accountant or attorney to help you with this and to help you plan for their future.

Gather together key documents and contact information that your family will need. Specific items you should consider are as follows:

- Attorney name and contact number.
- Executor of your estate and contact number.
- Legal documents (e.g., birth certificate, marriage certificate, divorce/separation papers, social security card, military records, power of attorney, and your will).
- Financial records (e.g., bank accounts, credit cards, investments, retirement and pension information, life insurance policies, deeds and titles to all property owned, mortgage, debts, and tax records).
- Health records (e.g., health insurance policies and advance directives; see Question 98).

You may feel troubled about unresolved issues in your life. If you have had a conflict with a close family member or friend, this might be the time to reach out and resolve your differences. If there is someone who has had a significant impact on your life, this might be the time to tell him or her how much the relationship has meant to you. If there is someone you love and perhaps have taken for granted, this might be the time to express your love for him or her. If you have belongings that are particularly precious, you may want to write out a list to indicate whom you would like to leave each of them to and include this in your will.

Some people find fulfillment in planning their own funeral. Your funeral should be a celebration of your life, and being involved in the details will ensure that it reflects all that you care about. Some specific suggestions include the following:

- Give your family a list of the people you would like to be invited to the service.
- Ask a clergy person with whom you have a personal relationship to officiate.
- Select particular passages to be read or particular pieces of music to be played that are meaningful to you.
- Choose special pictures or favorite flowers that you would like displayed.
- Decide on a particular funeral home, and consider whether you prefer a burial or cremation (you may even want to select a casket or urn).
- Select a particular cemetery if you want a burial.
- Choose a favorite outfit in which you would like to be buried.
- Write out things that you would like to have included in your obituary.

One thing that is particularly difficult to face is the thought of leaving loved ones (particularly children) behind, knowing you will no longer be a part of their lives after you have died. If you are concerned that you will die before your children or grandchildren have gotten to know you well, you may find it helpful to leave a part of yourself behind. Think about putting together an album of photos, writing out your life story, or making a video of yourself telling stories about key events in your life. If you feel sad that you will not be able to be present at some future important occasion, think about what you would want to say at that time and write a letter or narrate your thoughts on tape. This may be very meaningful to a child or grandchild at some time in the future—on the occasion of his or her marriage or at the birth of his or her own child.

100. Where can I get more information?

The Internet is becoming the most up-to-date source of information on cancer and its treatment. If you do not have a computer, a family member or friend, most local libraries, and most hospitals may have a computer that is available for your use.

Most of the Internet addresses listed here are the home pages of each organization. Spend time searching within each site to find specific information and to explore the other information and links that you find. Your time will be rewarded as you increase the knowledge and understanding of your disease and treatment and as you discover the numerous resources for information and support that are available to help you, your family, and your friends.

The Internet addresses listed later here are accurate as of March 2002; however, keep in mind that these addresses may change over time. Telephone numbers, if available, are listed with the Internet address.

Pancreatic Cancer Sites

Pancreatica
Web site: *www.pancreatica.org*
Provides information regarding clinical trials and other responsible medical care in the treatment of pancreatic cancer.

Pancreatic Cancer Action Network (PanCAN)
Phone: 1-877-2-PANCAN
Web site: *www.pancan.org*
Focuses national attention on the need to find a cure for pancreatic cancer (also provides links to sites with information on pancreatic cancer).

Lustgarten Foundation for Pancreatic Cancer Research
Phone: 1-866-789-1000
Web site: *www.lustgartenfoundation.org*
Enhances the science and medical research related to the diagnosis, treatment, cure, and prevention of pancreatic cancer (also provides links to sites with information on pancreatic cancer).

Cancer and Cancer Treatment

National Cancer Institute (NCI)
Chemotherapy and You: A Guide to Self Help During Treatment
Radiation Therapy and You: A Guide to Self Help During Treatment
Eating Hints for Cancer Patients: Before, During, and After Treatment
Phone: 1-800-4-CANCER (Cancer Information Service)
Web site: *www.nci.nih.gov*
Provides extensive information to patients and families.

American Cancer Society (ACS)
Phone: 1-800-ACS–2345
Web site: *www.cancer.org*
Provides information and support with links to community services.

National Comprehensive Cancer Network (NCCN)
Phone: 1-888-909-NCCN
Web site: *www.nccn.org*
An alliance of the worlds leading cancer centers that has developed treatment guidelines, an outcomes database, and links to other cancer-related sites.

The Cancer Information Network (CancerLinksUSA)
Web site: *www.thecancerinfo.org*
Provides information and links to other cancer-related sites.

Oncolink
Web site: *www.oncolink.com*
Sponsored by the University of Pennsylvania. Provides information on cancer, treatment, and clinical trials.

Johns Hopkins Pancreatic Cancer Home Page
Web site: *www.path.jhu.edu/pancreas*
Sponsored by the Johns Hopkins Medical Institutions. Provides information on pancreatic cancer, treatment, and clinical trials, and links to other cancer-related sites.

CancerWise
Web site: *www.cancerwise.org*
Sponsored by the University of Texas M. D. Anderson Cancer Center, a monthly electronic publication that contains information on cancer treatment and research. Can search previous issues for articles on pancreatic cancer.

Royal Marsden Hospital
Web site: *www.royalmarsden.org/patientinfo/booklets/index.asp*

CancerSource
Web site: *www.cancersource.com*
Provides information and support.

Symptom Management

National Cancer Institute (NCI)
Pain Control: A Guide for People with Cancer and Their Families
Phone: 1-800-4-CANCER (Cancer Information Service)
Web site: *www.nci.nih.gov*
Provides information for patients on managing a variety of symptoms, including pain and fatigue.

National Comprehensive Cancer Network (NCCN)
Phone: 1-888-909-NCCN
Web site: *www.nccn.org*
Provides guidelines for patients on managing pain, fatigue, and nausea, and vomiting.

Royal Marsden Hospital
Web site: *www.royalmarsden.org/patientinfo/booklets/index.asp*

Selecting a Cancer Center or Oncologist

National Cancer Institute-Designated Comprehensive Cancer Centers
Phone: 1-800-4-CANCER (Cancer Information Service)
Web site: *www.cancer.gov/clinical_trials/finding*
Web site (search by state):
  www.cancer.gov/clinical_trials/doc.aspx?viewid=b0d39c64-b8fd–415a-a778-bbe01257ace1
Provides a directory of centers recognized for scientific excellence and extensive cancer resources.

National Comprehensive Cancer Network (NCCN)
Phone: 1-888-909-6226
Web site: *www.nccn.org*
Provides a referral service of physicians specializing in the treatment of pancreatic cancer within the alliance of leading cancer centers.

Approved Hospital Cancer Program of the Commission on Cancer
Web site: *www.facs.org/public_info/yourhealth/aahcp.html*

Appendix

Provides a listing of hospitals that the American College of Surgeons approves of that can be searched by city, state, and category.

Association of Community Cancer Centers (ACCC)
Web site: *www.accc-cancer.org/members/map.html*
Provides a geographic listing of ACCC members with contact information and a description of cancer program and services.

American Board of Medical Specialties
Phone: 1-866-ASK-ABMS
Web site: *www.abms.org*
Provides verification of physician qualifications (who is certified).

American Medical Association
Phone: 1-312-464-5000
Web site: *www.ama-assn.org/aps/amahg.htm*
Maintains a database of demographic and professional information on individual physicians in the United States.

Clinical Trials

Pancreatica
Web site: *www.pancreatica.org*

Pancreatic Cancer Action Network (PanCAN)
Phone: 1-877-2-PANCAN
Web site: *www.pancan.org*

National Cancer Institute
Taking Part in Clinical Trials: What Cancer Patients Need to Know
Phone: 1-800-4-CANCER (Cancer Information Service)
Web site: *www.cancer.gov/clinical_trials*

National Institutes of Health
Web site: *clinicaltrials.gov*

Centerwatch
Phone: 1-617-856-5900
Web site: *www.centerwatch.com*

Coalition of National Cancer Cooperative Groups
Phone: 1-877-520-4457
Web site: *cancertrialshelp.org*

Complementary and Alternative Therapies

Cancer Information Service of the National Cancer Institute
Phone: 1-800-4-CANCER (Cancer Information Service)
Web site: *cis.nci.nih.gov/fact/9_14.htm*

National Center for Complementary and Alternative Medicine of the National Institutes of Health (NCCAM)
Phone: 1-888-644-6226
Web site: *nccam.nih.gov/*
Web site: *nccam.nih.gov/fcp/factsheets/index.html*
Web site: *nccam.nih.gov/fcp/faq/considercam.htm*

Oncolink (University of Pennsylvania)
Web site: *oncolink.upenn.edu/templates/treatment/index.cfm*

National Library of Medicine
Web site: *www.nlm.nih.gov/nccam/camonpubmed.html*

American Academy of Medical Acupuncture
Phone: 1-323-937-5514
Web site: *www.medicalacupuncture.org*

Dietary Supplements, including Vitamins, Minerals, and Botanicals

Office of Dietary Supplements of the National Institutes of Health
Web site: *dietary-supplements.info.nih.gov/databases/ibids.html*

Center for Food Safety and Applied Nutrition of the US Food and Drug Administration
Phone: 1-888-INFO-FDA
Web site: *www.cfsan.fda.gov*

American Botanical Council
Phone: 1-512-926-4900
Web site: *www.herbalgram.org*

Supplement Watch
Phone: 1-801-712-0408
Web site: *supplementwatch.com*

Quackwatch
Web site: *www.quackwatch.com*

Coping

National Cancer Institute (NCI)
Taking Time: Support for People With Cancer and the People Who Care About Them
When Cancer Recurs: Meeting the Challenge Again
Phone: 1-800-4-CANCER (Cancer Information Service)
Web site: *www.nci.nih.gov*

Cancer Care
Phone: 1-800-813-HOPE (4673)
Web site: *www.cancercare.org*

American Cancer Society (ACS)
Phone: 1-800-ACS–2345
Web site: *www.cancer.org*

National Coalition for Cancer Survivorship
Phone: 1-877-NCCS-YES
Web site: *www.cansearch.org* (under Programs, select Cancer Survivor Toolbox, an audio program on coping)

R. A. Bloch Cancer Foundation
Phone: 1-800-433-0464
Web site: *www.blochcancer.org*

Cancer Supportive Care Program
Web site: *www.cancersupportivecare.com*

Appearance and Sexuality

American Cancer Society Look Good, Feel Better program
Phone: 1-800-395-LOOK
Web site: *www.lookgoodfeelbetter.org*

American Association of Sex Educators, Counselors and Therapists
Web site: *www.aasect.org*

American Cancer Society (ACS)
Sexuality and Cancer: For the Woman Who Has Cancer, and Her Partner
Sexuality and Cancer: For the Man Who Has Cancer, and His Partner
Phone: 1-800-ACS-2345
Web site: *www.cancer.org*

Jacques Darcel, full-color catalogue of wigs for medical purposes
Phone: 1-212-753-7576

Ruth L. Weintraub Co. Inc., Buyer's Guide to Wigs and Hairpieces
Phone: 1-212-838-1333

Support Groups

(includes live and online groups, groups led by professionals, and one-on-one support)
Cancer Care
Phone: 1-800-813-HOPE (4673)
Web site: *www.cancercare.org*

Wellness Community
Phone: 1-888-793-WELL
Web site: *www.wellness-community.org*

Association of Cancer Online Resources
Web site: *www.acor.org*

Appendix

Cancer Hope Network
Phone: 1-877-HOPENET
Web site: *www.cancerhopenetwork.org*

OncoChat
Web site: *www.oncochat.org*

Gilda's Club
Phone: 1-917-305-1200
Web site: *www.gildasclub.org*

R. A. Bloch Cancer Foundation
Web site: *www.blochcancer.org*

Caregivers

National Family Caregivers Association
Phone: 1-800-896-3650
Web site: *www.nfcacares.org*

American Cancer Society (ACS)
Caregiving: A Step-By-Step Resource for Caring for the Person with Cancer at Home
Phone: 1-800-ACS–2345
Web site: *www.cancer.org*

National Coalition for Cancer Survivorship
Phone: 1-877-NCCS-YES
Web site: *www.cansearch.org* (under Programs, select Caring for the Caregiver, an audio program)

Speaking with Children
When a Parent is Sick: Helping Parents Explain Serious Illness to Children, by Joan Hamilton, published by Pottersfield Press through Nimbus Publishing (ISBN 1-895-900-40-9)
Phone: 1-800-NIMBUS–9 (1-800-646-2879)

National Cancer Institute
When Someone in Your Family Has Cancer
Phone: 1-800-4-CANCER (Cancer Information Service)
Web site: *www.nci.nih.gov*

KidsCope (Web site designed to help children understand and deal with the effects of cancer on a parent)
Web site: *www.kidscope.org*

Financial Support

American Cancer Society (ACS)
Phone: 1-800-ACS–2345
Web site: *www.cancer.org*

Cancer Care
Phone: 1-800-813-HOPE (4673)
Web site: *www.cancercare.org*

Health Insurance Association of America (HIAA)
Phone: 1-202-824-1600
Web site: *www.hiaa.org*

Certified Financial Planner Board of Standards
Phone: 1-888-CFP-MARK
Web site: *www.cfp-board.org*

Financial Planning Association
Phone: 1-800-282-7526
Web site: *www.fpanet.org*

Social Security Administration Office of Public Inquiries
Phone: 1-800-772-1213
Phone: 1-800-325-0778 (TTY)
Web site: *www.ssa.gov*

Centers for Medicare and Medicaid Services
Web site: *ww.hcfa.gov*

Department of Veterans Affairs
Phone: 1-202-273-5400 (Washington, D.C. office)
Phone: 1-800-827-1000 (local VA office)
Web site: *www.va.gov*
Provides information about benefits for those who have served in the armed forces.

Appendix

Health Resources and Services Administration
Phone: 1-800-638-0742
Phone: 1-800-492-0359 (if calling from Maryland)
Web site: *www.hrsa.gov/osp/dfcr/about/aboutdiv.htm*
Provides information about the Hill-Burton Program, in which
designated hospitals provide free or low-cost care.

Financial Assistance for Prescription Drugs

Cancer Care
Phone: 1-800-813-HOPE (4673)
Web site: *www.cancercare.org/hhrd/drug_assistance.asp*

Cancer Supportive Care Program
Web site: *www.cancersupportivecare.com/pharmacy.html*

NeedyMeds
Phone: 1-215-625-9609
Web site: *www.needymeds.com*

Legal Issues

Family and Medical Leave Act
United States Department of Labor
Web site: *www.dol.gov/dol/esa/public/regs/statutes/whd/fmla.htm*
Web site: *www.dol.gov/dol/esa/fmla.htm*

Americans with Disabilities Act
U.S. Department of Justice
Phone: 1-800-514-0301
Web site: *www.usdoj.gov/crt/ada/adahom1.htm*
U.S. Equal Employment Opportunity Commission (EEOC):
federal laws prohibiting job discrimination
Phone: 1-202-663-4900
Web site: *www.eeoc.gov*

End of Life

National Cancer Institute (NCI)
Advanced Cancer: Living Each Day
Phone 1-800-4-CANCER (Cancer Information Service)
Web site: *www.nci.nih.gov*

Partnership for Caring
Phone: 1-800-989-9455
Web site: *www.partnershipforcaring.org*
Provides information on end of life issues, including advance
   directives.

Last Acts
Web site: *www.lastacts.org*
Provides information on end of life issues.

National Hospice and Palliative Care Organization
Phone: 1-800-658-8898
Web site: *www.nhpco.org*
Provides listing of local hospices.

National Hospice Foundation
Phone: 1-800-338-8619
Web site: *www.hospiceinfo.org*
Provides information to help in selecting a hospice.

Hospice Net
Web site: *www.hospicenet.org*
Provides information for patients and caregivers on end of life
   issues and bereavement.

Appendix

Glossary

Acupuncture: a treatment adapted from Chinese medical practice that involves placement of needles at precise points on the body that are believed to connect with pathways that relieve pain or produce local anesthesia.

Adjuvant therapy: use of chemotherapy, radiation therapy, or both following surgical removal of a malignant tumor; adjuvant treatment is used to try to prevent recurrence of cancer.

Analgesics: medications to relieve pain.

Anemia: low red blood cell counts.

Antioxidants: chemical substances that may protect your cells against the effects of certain compounds (free radicals), which can cause cell damage.

Ascites: abnormal build up of fluid in the abdominal cavity, generally related to cancer.

Bilirubin: substance produced in the liver when the body breaks down hemoglobin, the molecule in red blood cells that carries oxygen; it is yellowish green in color and is eliminated in bile.

Bone marrow: substance in the center of many bones, including the ribs, long bones of the legs, and vertebrae, where blood cells are produced.

Cancerous: malignant, capable of invading tissue and spreading to distant organs.

Celiac axis: network of nerves in the upper abdomen adjacent to the pancreas.

Cells: the smallest structural unit of a living organism.

Chemoradiotherapy: treatment consisting of a combination of chemotherapy and radiation therapy, also termed combined modality therapy.

Chemotherapy: medications generally given either intravenously or orally to destroy cancer cells.

Clinical trial: research study to test a new treatment on human subjects.

Complementary therapy: a variety of approaches to improve health and treat disease that are not recognized as standard by the traditional medical community but that are used in addition to standard methods of treatment, e.g. acupuncture, homeopathy.

Complete response: disappearance of all signs of disease as a result of treatment.

Computed tomography (CT) scan: a diagnostic test that uses a x-rays and a computer system to create detailed images of structures inside the body.

Contrast media: a substance given by mouth or by injection into a vein to provide better visualization of a particular organ on an x-ray or CT scan.

Deep vein thrombosis: presence of a blood clot in a deep vein, typically in the calf.

Differentiation: specialization in appearance and function.

Endocrine: gland that secretes substances directly into the blood stream.

Endoscopic retrograde cholangiopancreatogram (ERCP): procedure done to evaluate the liver, gallbladder, bile ducts, and pancreas; a flexible lighted tube (endoscope) is passed through the mouth, esophagus, stomach, and upper intestine to the point where the duct from the pancreas and gallbladder drains into the intestine. A catheter is inserted into the duct and contrast media is injected so the ducts can be seen on an x-ray; if abnormal growths are seen, an instrument can be passed through the tube and used to take a sample of tissue (biopsy) for examination under the microscope.

Endoscopy: procedure for examining the inside of a body tube or of a hollow organ.

Exocrine: gland that secretes substances through a duct.

External beam radiation therapy: radiation therapy administered by a machine in which a beam of radiation is directed to a defined part of the body.

Genetic: affected by genes, parts of chromosomes which influence the structure or function of the body.

Healthcare proxy: a health care surrogate, a medical proxy, or a medical power of attorney; a person authorized to make health care decisions for you if you are not in a position to do so.

Hereditary: passed on through the genes from one generation to the next.

Integrative medicine: the use of complementary or alternative therapies, a variety of approaches to improve health and treat disease that are not recognized as standard by the traditional medical community.

Intraoperative radiation therapy (IORT): administration of radiation therapy at the time of surgery.

Intravenously: through a vein.

Jaundice: yellowing of the skin or eyes from a build up of bilirubin in the blood stream and skin.

Locally advanced pancreatic cancer: stage of pancreatic cancer in which the tumor has invaded local tissues or is closely wrapped around vital structures, such as major blood vessels; can not be surgically removed.

Lymphatic channels: vessels throughout the body that drain lymph fluid.

Magnetic resonance imaging (MRI): a diagnostic test that uses a large magnet, radio waves, and a computer system to create detailed images of structures inside the body.

Margins: the edges of any tissue removed by surgery.

Mediport: device implanted under the skin with a connecting catheter that is threaded into a large vein in the chest; provides a way to draw blood and administer chemotherapy.

Metabolism: the physical and chemical processes required to maintain life.

Metastasis: spread of a malignant tumor to a distant organ.

Migratory thrombophlebitis: formation of blood clots in the superficial veins of the arms or legs.

Mutations: abnormal alteration in the structure of the DNA molecule (gene).

Nerve block: injection of alcohol or a painkilling medication into a mass of nerves to relieve pain.

Oncologists: physicians specializing in the treatment of cancer; generally further specialized as medical, surgical, or radiation therapy oncologists.

Palliative: to relieve symptoms.

Pancreatic insufficiency: inability of the pancreas to secrete an adequate amount of enzymes needed to digest food.

Paracentesis: procedure to drain fluid (ascites) that has built up in the abdominal cavity.

Partial response: decrease in the size of a tumor, by at least 50%, as a result of treatment.

Performance status: level of functioning that is scored based on a person's activity during the day and ability to care for him- or herself.

Platelet: blood cells that stop bleeding by clumping together to plug a damaged blood vessel.

Prognosis: the most likely outcome of a disease.

Progression: growth of a tumor or spread of a tumor to a distant site in the body.

Simulation: procedure that is part of the planning process for the administration of radiation therapy; involves x-rays or CT scans to identify the area to be treated and tattooing the skin to ensure correct positioning each day of treatment.

Spleen: an organ in the upper left side of the abdomen that serves to filter the blood.

Stable disease: no growth of a tumor; considered a favorable situation for patients with pancreatic cancer.

Stereotactic radiation: administration of radiation therapy using special devices to pinpoint the beam of radiation to a small precisely defined region of the body.

Steroid: a category of medication with many different uses; most often used to reduce an inflammatory response.

Stomatitis: inflammation of the mucous membranes of the mouth from chemotherapy; may be associated with sores, ulcers, and mouth pain. Also called **mucositis**.

Surgical bypass: surgical procedure used when there is a blockage, to create an alternative passage for body substances.

Tumor: abnormal growth, can be cancerous (malignant) or noncancerous (benign).

Tumor markers: substances produced by malignant tumors that can be measured in the blood.

Ultrasound: a diagnostic test that uses sound waves to create images of structures inside the body.

Venous thrombosis: presence of a blood clot in a vein.

Whipple surgery: surgical removal of the head of the pancreas, the upper end of the duodenum, and the lower end of the bile duct; also involves reconnecting the stomach, the bile duct, and the pancreatic duct to the small intestine.

White blood cells: a variety of blood cells that fight infection.

Index

Index